HOMEOPATHY

Gillian Stokes

TEACH YOURSELF BOOKS

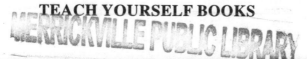

The author acknowledges the help and support of James Pellicott, who provided the original ideas for the illustrations.

For UK orders: please contact Bookpoint Ltd, 39 Milton Park, Abingdon, Oxon OX14 4TD. Telephone: (44) 01235 400414, Fax: (44) 01235 400454. Lines are open from 9.00–6.00, Monday to Saturday, with a 24 hour message answering service. Email address: orders@bookpoint.co.uk

For USA & Canada orders: please contact NTC/Contemporary Publishing, 4255 West Touhy Avenue, Lincolnwood, Illinois 60646–1975, USA. Telephone: (847) 679 5500, Fax: (847) 679 2494.

Long renowned as the authoritative source for self-guided learning – with more than 30 million copies sold worldwide – the *Teach Yourself* series includes over 200 titles in the fields of languages, crafts, hobbies, business and education.

British Library Cataloguing in Publication Data
A catalogue entry for this title is available from The British Library.

Library of Congress Catalog Card Number: On file

First published in UK 1999 by Hodder Headline Plc, 338 Euston Road, London, NW1 3BH.

First published in US 1999 by NTC/Contemporary Publishing, 4255 West Touhy Avenue, Lincolnwood (Chicago), Illinois 60646–1975 USA.

The 'Teach Yourself' name and logo are registered trade marks of Hodder & Stoughton Ltd.

Copyright © 1999 Gillian Stokes

Typeset by Transet Limited, Coventry, England.
Printed in Great Britain for Hodder & Stoughton Educational, a division of Hodder Headline Plc, 338 Euston Road, London NW1 3BH by Cox & Wyman Ltd, Reading, Berkshire.

Impression number   10 9 8 7 6 5 4 3 2
Year   2004 2003 2002 2001 2000 1999

CONTENTS

The highest ideal of therapy is to restore health rapidly, gently, permanently; to remove and destroy the whole disease in the shortest, surest, least harmful way, according to clearly comprehensible principles.

Samuel Hahnemann: *The Organon of the Healing Art*

AN INTRODUCTION
TO HOMEOPATHY

Similia similibus curentur: let like be cured with like

What is homeopathy?

Homeopathy is a natural, holistic complement to conventional, or allopathic, medicine. Homeopathy works with the body's own healing system, treating the person, not a disease. A healing response is triggered by administering a minute amount of the same substance which would provoke the problematic symptoms if taken by a healthy person. Given as a tiny, potentized remedy it stimulates the body's natural response – what Hahnemann called the will to health, or vital force – to effect self cure. All homeopathic treatment is by means of pharmacological prescribing, according to strict rules and principles.

The idea of a vital force with the power to heal is known in other belief systems, such as the Hindu *Prāna*, the ancient Greek *Pneuma*, and the Chinese *Ch'i*. The idea of an invisible, intelligent healing force may seem unlikely to Western thought, but we should remember how many other natural and invisible regulatory processes we accept without question; the hormonal system; generic DNA; the autonomic nervous system; the auto-immune system; and so on. As with the vital force, we can observe the results of these processes at work, but not the controlling force behind them. That homeopathically prepared remedies may exert an influence to stimulate health, perhaps upon the body's energy patterns, does not seem to be beyond the bounds of possibility. Indeed many other healing treatments which have gained the respect of patients and conventional medical practitioners alike, such as acupuncture, also assume the existence and influence upon the body of invisible channels or fields of energy.

Homeopathy is not a new age fad. The basic principle of treating like with like to strengthen the body's own defence was known in ancient Greece but was tested, extended and systematized by Samuel Hahnemann in Europe almost two hundred years ago. Hahnemann formulated a strict set of rules and codes of practice which have been applied by classical homeopaths ever since. This gentle healing art is now widely practised throughout the world.

Homeopathy: training and control

There are carefully trained and certified practitioners all around the world. Professional homeopaths in Britain undergo a rigorous training which includes expert knowledge of anatomy and physiology. Many British homeopaths are also fully trained and qualified in conventional medicine; as general practitioners, pharmacists, physicians and surgeons. Believing in the efficacy of homeopathy, they have decided to undertake the demanding additional training necessary for accreditation by The British Homoeopathic Association. This is the British homeopathic governing body which confers the status MFHom upon suitably qualified medical practitioners. The Society of Homoeopaths confers RSHom accreditation upon professionally qualified homeopaths who do not also have conventional medical qualifications, other than the anatomy and physiology which are core components of all serious homeopathic study. Tremendous levels of dedication, commitment and study are thus required of accredited homeopaths, and despite the extra time, effort and expense required to gain accreditation, there is a worldwide expansion of interest, especially in South America.

In the United States of America any homeopathic doctor must first train with an allopathic medical school, and pass the same examinations as a conventional doctor before undertaking additional homeopathic training. All American homeopathic products are also legally required to be regulated in the same way as allopathic drugs. (In each case a National Drug Code number must be clearly displayed, to verify that the product is Food and Drug Administration (FDA) approved, and has been made in accordance with the regulations for all medicines within the US

Homeopathic Pharmacopoeia.) Homeopathic remedies may legally be sold without a doctor's prescription in the United States and in Great Britain.

France has long accepted homeopathy as an alternative to allopathy and most pharmacists offer both treatments. Remedy potencies are restricted to low dosages by Napoleonic law and this has led to some differences in French prescribing techniques. In France each strength or potency of the same remedy may be prescribed as if it was a different remedy, and remedies are often given in combination. Both of these practices conflict with original, classical homeopathy as defined by Hahnemann. There is nevertheless widespread respect for homeopathy in France, and remedies are well made and cheap to buy.

Germany, as may be expected of the birthplace of homeopathy, has very many practitioners and training schools. German homeopaths also favour the practice of combining remedies, counter to Hahnemann's classical homeopathic methodology.

The Indian subcontinent has a long tradition of employing homeopathic philosophy and practice. Formal training in India has produced a huge number of registered homeopaths. (Of course, Hindus take remedies prepared in different ways because sac lac tablets are products of the cow.) Many textbooks written by Hahnemann and his followers, and used by students worldwide today, originated in Indian publishing houses. Practitioners with less formal training methodologies may be no less adept practitioners of homeopathy. Many have a long-standing cultural history of favouring homeopathic principles rather than orthodoxy, and adhere to the same essential principles which govern homeopathic prescribing anywhere. Any absence of certification may be compensated for by the greater wealth of experience.

Why choose homeopathy?

A gentle treatment

Homeopathy is a gentle and effective healing art; an art which applies scientifically valid, empirically tested practices. Classically trained homeopathic practitioners select remedies according to rules and principles which have been tried, tested and unchanged for almost two hundred years. By influencing the patient's own energy patterns, homeopathically prepared remedies gently encourage the body to restore healthy equilibrium. Typically, each homeopathic remedy is given singly in the minimum number of applications possible, to produce a response. This allows for uncomplicated treatment, and for the accurate monitoring of results. The remedy can then be withdrawn as soon as the healing response is noted, or an adjustment to a different remedy made, if necessary.

Conventional medical treatments attack symptoms, which to the homeopath are merely evidence of the body's fight against dis-ease. Unfortunately many conventional (or allopathic) drugs also have a harsh effect on the body causing new iatrogenic symptoms (side effects) which then require alleviation with further medication. It is not uncommon for chronically ill patients to be taking a number of allopathic pills and potions daily, making any assessment of the effects of any single medicine difficult, and masking any healing response to the original problem. Some allopathic medicines may appear to remove unwanted symptoms successfully, but homeopaths believe they may do so merely by driving the root problem deeper within the body, causing more critical damage which may not surface for many years.

Ease of use

Children, and adults who find swallowing pills difficult, will be pleased to know that homeopathic pills are tiny and dissolve under the tongue, without an unpleasant taste. If administering these is still too difficult, as it may be with an infant or an animal, the remedy may be prescribed in the form of a tasteless, or slightly sweet, liquid rather than a tablet. This can be added to drinking water.

No animal testing

The welfare of animals might be a reason for some people to choose homeopathy. Though some homeopathic remedies are prepared from animal source materials, the remedies are not tested on animals. For homeopathic proving purposes it would be pointless if they were, since objective and subjective reporting of clinical experience are both essential. A horse cannot communicate that it experienced a tingling in its near, hind hoof, felt a strong desire to eat apples, and had thoughts of rolling in long grass after taking a remedy; and even if it could, it is doubtful how accurate or useful a human correlation of that expression would be. We can never know how another species experiences the world, beyond inferring suppositions from observed behaviour, and should not assume there would be human similarity of response. Of course in treating animals homeopathically it is possible to observe and infer, but this is not adequate for determining the effects of, or *proving*, a remedy for inclusion in a human Materia Medica. However, homeopathic remedies are thoroughly tested. Willing human volunteers continue to add to the body of knowledge, by bravely testing new substances, and confirming old ones, as did Hahnemann throughout his homeopathic career. Subjective reporting is an essential aspect of proving a homeopathic remedy.

Allopathic dissatisfactions

Homeopathy is enjoying a resurgence today due in part to dissatisfaction with conventional methodology and also as more and more people describe to their friends the positive benefits they have experienced. Some patients receiving conventional treatment under the British NHS care system express disquiet at the short time allotted for a medical appointment, usually a scant ten minutes or so per patient. Doubt arises whether a meaningful diagnosis can be made with such a rapid throughput of patients per surgery, or few minutes per home visit, as it is necessary to see the maximum number of patients per day. Time is money and professional time is more money. In defence it may be argued that pressure of work dictates such strictures, but patients increasingly express doubts as to how meaningful such a short assessment of their medical case and life circumstances can be, as the basis for determining an appropriate treatment for their condition. If conventional doctors allotted as much time per patient as the homeopath must, far fewer patients could be seen per day, per doctor, with an attendant drop in income, unless charges rose steeply to compensate for the reduced caseload.

The changing faces of medicine

It has also become unusual for a patient to remain with a single doctor for a lifetime and one may rarely see the same doctor twice. Patients move, doctors move, hospitals close down, and imperfect records and recollections are all that informs the conventional doctor at each new and brief consultation, if indeed past records are available at all. The homeopath must expend more time and intellectual effort with the patient than the conventional doctor is likely to be able to. Classical homeopathic methodology demands that this be so, to discover the remedy best suited to you, as an individual, with your life history, as you are today. The homeopath's basic methodology requires professional involvement and expertise in all aspects of assessment and treatment throughout the healthcare, which makes delegation impractical and counterproductive. All preliminary and subsequent casetaking interviews, all subsequent treatment, prescribing and checking of results, will therefore normally be undertaken by the professional homeopath in person. Nowadays the allopathic practitioner increasingly delegates many of these tasks to less trained healthcare workers, such as nurses or paramedics. This delegation is a sensible conservation of the doctor's valuable professional time which can then be deployed where greater expertise is essential, but the patient may find the consistent attentiveness offered by the homeopath more appealing.

Royal approval

Homeopathy has been used and supported by many members of the British Royal family ever since it was introduced early in the nineteenth century by the consort of William IV, Queen Adelaide. Among the current Royal family Her Majesty, Queen Elizabeth II, and Charles, Prince of Wales are known to have taken homeopathic advice regularly. Her Majesty the Queen is said to travel with a box of homeopathic remedies, and to employ a consultant homeopath when necessary. Prince Charles is an outspoken advocate for homeopathy and other complementary treatments.

Allopathy and homeopathy: different treatment approaches

Conventional (allopathic) medicine and homeopathy take different approaches to healing. Allopathy aims to counteract symptoms. It assumes the body is constantly threatened by invaders, such as bacteria and viruses, which compromise health and well being. These must be repelled if the symptoms of illness are to be alleviated, so conventional medicines are designed to attack, and rid the body of such invaders; removing, reversing, or suppressing symptoms in various ways. Many conventional medicines work on the justification principle of the greater good; accepting that undesirable additional effects or risks may attend their use. So, we will be given antacids for stomach acidity, antihistamines to reverse a histamine reaction, and antibiotics to quell all bacteria, whether useful or harmful. Conventional medicine also regards pathology as of great importance; the idea that collections of symptoms form an identifiable dis-ease, although which pathological indicators have been considered significant has changed frequently throughout medical history. Homeopathy, in contrast, does not attack the symptom manifestations of imbalance but uses them as a guide to effective stimulation of the vital force.

Allopathic health is thus to be symptom free; but achieving this may involve long term use of counteractive medicines, which often introduce unwelcome risks and side effects. Health to a homeopath is a well-balanced organism which is able to shrug off stress when it is encountered, whether the stress is physical, mental, emotional or environmental, in order to maintain a balanced state of health. Correction of any imbalance is typically achieved by administering a single remedy of the lowest possible potency, for the shortest time required to trigger a healing response. Viruses and bacteria are acknowledged by homeopaths, but are believed to have little or no effect upon the vital force of a strong and healthy body exposed to them. We know that meningococcal bacteria are present in the throats of a very large proportion of the population for example, yet outbreaks of the disease, meningitis, are rare.

Symptoms, to the homeopathic way of thinking, are evidence of how the body is mounting its own defence, and in order to restore health, symptoms should be noted and enabled, not repressed or attacked. To the homeopath, symptoms are part of the cure, they are not the dis-ease. Pathology is not ignored, however; familiar descriptive terms can be an aid to communication, and are useful if prescribing for acute, first-aid situations, but pathology is not the classical homeopathic basis for the selection of a remedy.

Scientific homeopathy

Homeopathy has been accused of being unscientific but it is quite as scientific as allopathy, even by orthodoxy's own terms of reference. After all, the conventional (allopathic) doctor abandons the scientific model when making a diagnosis, and again when prescribing, according to science's own defining criteria. The patient may have undergone all manner of pathological tests and procedures, all properly scientific, but the diagnosis the doctor infers from the results, and the decision of what to prescribe, still rely upon his or her less scientific personal, subjective experience, training and intuition. When treating, the orthodox doctor must also consider the ever-changing treatments and medications available. How well he or she does so varies according to available time and willingness to keep abreast of change. Different allopathic doctors favour different diagnostic tests, and reach different conclusions even if presented with the results from the same tests. Most professional homeopaths if presented with the same complexity of symptoms, would suggest the same single matching remedy and would have done so at any time during the history of homeopathy. Symptom picture do not alter over time. The Materia Medica has been extended with the proving of new substances but the original ones have remained as true a picture of symptoms today as ever. So, as a stick to beat homeopathy, science does not always serve its orthodox master well, but until an explanation for homeopathy is found which is acceptable to scientists, the debate will continue, and it is good that it should. Any medical practice must be open to critical appraisal; but we should not automatically condemn what cannot be explained.

There is an allopathic assumption of universally identifiable diseases, recognized from patterns of symptoms (pathology). Conventional medicine (allopathy) identifies these named diseases, aided by laboratory tests and technological diagnostic equipment, from the general symptoms presented.	In contrast, homeopathy sees symptoms as evidence of an innate will to health, which manifests uniquely in each person. The well-trained homeopath identifies the unique evidence of the healing impulse in each person, rather than grouping together those persons with some common symptom similarities and labelling them as victims of a common disease to be given the identical remedy. Even the homeopath who treats acute symptoms will use homeopathic principles in selecting the correct remedy for the individual who has this or that common condition.
There is an underlying allopathic assumption that disease is caused by intervention from outside, and intervention from outside effects a cure. The allopathic treatment of disease therefore employs medicines which produce the opposite effect to the troubling symptoms, or which overpower, suppress or eradicate them.	The homeopathic view of symptoms is that they are evidence of the body's effort to restore health following exposure to stress of one kind or another. If the vital force which encountered the stress had not been weakened, there would have been no imbalance, and no disease. The body's own regulatory system would have compensated less dramatically to maintain order; which is why we do not all fall ill when exposed to the same external influence.
To the conventional (allopathic) practitioner, individual symptoms are secondary in importance to pathology yet the importance attached to named pathological signs has varied throughout the history of medicine. In conventional medicine there is no coherent principle of what defines illness or health, nor any systematized definition of what constitutes a beneficial or harmful symptom, so the practitioner's interpretations are necessarily somewhat arbitrary.	However, the individual symptom indicators for proven homeopathic remedies have remained so accurate there has been no need to change them in almost two hundred years. The reliability of the original provings has been confirmed whenever remedies have been re-proved in recent years. Pathology is acknowledged in homeopathy, especially when prescribing for acute, first-aid situations, but the remedy is always selected to match individual symptoms, not merely according to overall pathology.

Figure 1   Homeopathic and allopathic philosophies compared

What can homeopathy treat?

Any loss of well being, whether physical, mental, emotional or constitutional, can be treated homeopathically. What is more, you need not wait to become ill to benefit from homeopathy. Impending life changes such as the menopause can be managed homeopathically according to your constitutional type, thus helping to avoid malaise before it is experienced. Social and environmental difficulties, beyond the normal scope of conventional medicine, can also be managed homeopathically.

Serious conditions can be treated in homeopathic hospitals either in conjunction with conventional treatments, or exclusively homeopathically, according to choice or necessity. Homeopathy can speedily aid recovery from surgical intervention, and undo ill effects caused by allopathic medicines, or vaccinations (iatrogenic symptoms). Chronic conditions such as asthma, eczema and hay fever seem to respond especially well to homeopathic treatment in the hands of a professional; often when the best efforts of conventional treatments have failed. Chronic conditions should only be treated by professional homeopaths, however, because they are deep-seated and often complicated by years of conventional intervention. The professional homeopath will need to draw out the original source of a chronic condition via several stages, as they were suppressed over the years, with different remedies given as each stage re-emerges, like the layers of an onion. Such skilled assessment and prescribing is not for the amateur, and is certainly beyond the intended scope of this book.

In contrast, acute conditions are temporary in nature and sudden in onset. They usually disappear equally quickly. Accidental injuries can respond well to homeopathic first aid, though common sense should dictate when to call in emergency professional help. Once help is on the way there is no harm in alleviating suffering with a well-chosen homeopathic remedy, if the patient welcomes it. Remember you have no right to insist on treating someone who does not want homeopathic intervention, however sure you may be that it would benefit them. The remedies in this book are intended for use with acute conditions and minor accidents only. The Materia Medica and Repertory have been selected with this in mind. The serious student would be well advised to obtain larger volumes of these works which encompass all known remedies and symptoms and to learn to practise classical homeopathy. Such books are available by mail as well as in specialist shops.

Animal treatments

Animals can be treated homeopathically, often with great success, despite their inability to relate their subjective experience to us. Indeed there are many veterinarians who combine homeopathy with their usual treatments, or treat exclusively in this way. So many observations have been made, one can now buy Repertories and Materia Medica based on observed animal symptoms, reports of the treatments, and noted reactions to remedies.

How does homeopathy work?

The honest answer is that no one knows, though there are many theories, ancient and modern. That it does work has been scientically and statistically documented, however. Homeopaths the world over have settled for that, while waiting for science to find the explanation. Medical trials are the focus for heated debates between those who can accept homeopathy based on practical results, and those who will not accept any result unless it is preceded by scientific explanations. There is no known mechanism for how homeopathic microdoses work, that is true, but neither is there a scientific explanation for how aspirin works when allopathically prescribed. Fortunately, lack of confirming theoretical evidence does not stop the widespread use and acceptance of aspirin, based on its observed benefits.

Homeopathy mistaken for vaccination

Homeopathy is often mistakenly described as similar to vaccination, in which a substance is directly introduced into the body by injection. Vaccination amounts to an unnatural assault on the body and overrides natural defence systems. The introduction of tiny amounts of vaccine (made from small quantities of live or dead disease material) is intended to elicit an antibody reaction. Vaccines trick the body's immune system into reacting as though it were really under attack. It is this which some mistakenly say makes vaccination like homeopathy, yet the same measured dose of vaccine is given to everyone, unlike the individually selected homeopathic remedy. Direct injections stress the body; homeopathic remedies do not. Homeopathy selects the remedy best suited to the individual, and the potency best suited to the severity of that person's condition, and introduces its material through the normal digestive system, with all its evolved systems of defence. Vaccination introduces the same substance, rather than a potentized agent known to produce like symptoms, and despite the fact that vaccines are prepared and tested by using animals and humans, it is still common for them to trigger unpleasant, and even life-threatening side effects. Currently the Measles, Mumps and Rubella combined booster vaccination is under investigation as a possible causal factor in Crohn's disease, the lifelong condition which causes great pain and discomfort.

The individualized remedy

The classical homeopath assesses all aspects of an individual to ascertain the root of the imbalance rather than isolates a named disease with only local effect. Everything about the individual will be taken into consideration, mind, body and soul, since the homeopath believes that the whole person manifests signs of reaction to a disease stimulus. Since there are no localized disease conditions, according to homeopathy, there can never be more than one reactive condition present in a person at any one time. Multiple symptoms will therefore be the various signs which collectively point to a single reaction process, and which by their nature also identify the remedy capable of assisting the body in its effort to restore health. This is so important I shall repeat it: *There is only one reactive condition present in a person at any one time. Multiple symptoms are the various signs which collectively point to a single reaction process, and which by their nature identify the remedy capable of assisting the body in its effort to restore health.*

The combination of factors which the classical homeopath will gather from observation and enquiry, amount to the personal characteristics which form an individual. For each individual what is normal is unique, and dis-ease is also a different experience than it would be for anyone else. No two people have the same dis-ease because no one is ill in an identical way. The classical homeopath will therefore enquire about the mental, emotional, genetic, environmental, and physical background, to discover what is normal for this person, and seek out what is currently peculiar or unusual. In this way the homeopath can build up a wide picture of the factors affecting the individual, the symptoms being experienced, and what would represent a healthy state of balance for him or her. A homeopathic remedy is prepared from a substance selected for a known and tested ability to produce, in a well person, symptoms similar to those being experienced by an individual patient as dis-ease. It is the patient's least common symptoms which are of interest to the homeopath, as these help to distinguish one potential remedy picture from another. (The allopath seeks similarities of symptoms according to pathological definitions.) Mental and emotional states are regarded as of greater importance than physical symptoms such as a headache or stomach ache. To the homeopath the inner state and sense of well-being are better measures of health and balance than physical symptoms, and may reveal the first sign of cure.

The holistic approach

The classical homeopathic method involves a painstaking assessment of the patient – of the patient, not of the disease. Nonetheless, it is common to speak of a condition or a complaint as if it were a universal, because we could not reasonably discuss long lists of symptoms and experiences, and because we are more familiar with allopathic generalities. Indeed many homeopaths treat for pathological conditions symptomatically, rather than for constitutional types. Patients, used to this approach with conventional medicine, have come to expect a cure for the specific symptoms for which they have consulted. Even so, the selection of the remedy will still be according to the strict homeopathic principles of matching symptoms to a single proved remedy, and the potency will still be the minimum to effect a healing response.

The difference is that what is prescribed will not necessarily be according to the underlying constitutional type. Even classical homeopaths may need to treat pathologically in emergency situations, where it is not possible to take the full case details properly. In this situation a remedy will be given which experience has shown to suit many people in similar circumstances, with similar symptoms. An example is the common practice of giving Arnica (internally) following a fright or sudden injury. However, the same cause may produce different symptoms, in different individuals, and then even in an emergency, a different remedy would be selected.

Whichever method of treatment is employed, the homeopath should always remain attentive and aware of the unique combination of symptoms which *this* individual is expressing, albeit within the broad description given to the condition. The correct remedy has to reflect the unique experience of the individual, as identified by what differs from a typical case, not by what makes it the same. It is not enough to treat all conditions which have a broadly similar picture with the same remedy (though treating acute conditions may in practice often involve using the same few remedies). For example, conventional medicine might say two people who each have a chest infection should be treated with an antibiotic. To treat them homeopathically, if one has a dry, unproductive cough, feels irritable and fidgety, worse at nights and feels better for fresh air; while the other produces copious amounts of phlegm, is lethargic and benefits from warmth, with the avoidance of draughts; their symptoms, and the most suitable homeopathic remedy, will differ, though in both cases the problem is a chest infection. Both could be said to have a cough, for the purposes of sensible communication, but their symptom picture and therefore remedy picture are wildly different.

So, it is helpful to think of the remedies as sets of symptoms, not as the antidotes of specific diseases. As you become more adept at recognizing the matching symptom pictures of the patients you treat, you will come to recognize remedy characteristics, the unusual, defining aspects of a remedy, when you encounter them, and will come to know them as such in your medicine cabinet. Thus it is the symptoms you will come to know, and the potentized remedy will treat them homeopathically only when it is a good individualized match.

Constitutional remedies

Constitutional prescribing, the province of the professional, recognizes and responds to the innate qualities expressed by a person when enjoying what, for them, is normal health. So, you might recognize a Phosphorus type at the bus stop, and the Sulphur type who you work alongside. The constitutional picture is helpful when presented with someone who describes a recent onset of symptoms which would not normally be true of them. It is not noteworthy that the person with a craving for spicy foods always has had a strong desire to eat curry, but it might be if normally they have an aversion to it. Constitutional homeopathic treatment when practised by a professional addresses the roots of chronic dis-ease.

Homeopathic treatment is thus of individuals (not of diseases) by means of matching a symptom-inducing substance, with observed

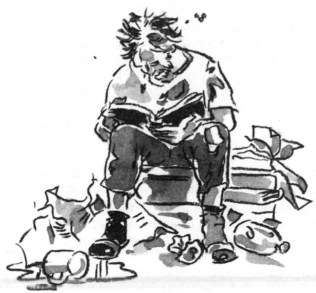

Figure 2   A sulphur constitutional type

symptoms. Each experience of disease is unique, even if some symptoms do seem to occur commonly. There is an underlying homeopathic assumption that the body will heal itself, if its vital force is stimulated to do so.

Symptomatic prescribing for acute situations (First Aid)

All first aid and minor injury problems share some similarities. These are the acute conditions. Often in such instances of acute disease a common symptom picture and common remedy may seem to apply which makes amateur treatment easier. There is a range of such illnesses, mental and physical, which may be treated on a first-aid basis. All will have had a sudden onset (incubation/accident); followed by a fairly predictable sequence of symptoms (acute); then symptoms vanish as the body restores control and equilibrium (convalescent). These are not life-threatening situations and usually respond well to routine prescribing at a 6C or 12C potency, which can safely be repeated (see Chapter 4 for more on potencies). Prescribing for an acute condition in this way is not like the classical homeopathy which addresses the patient's constitutional type, but circumstances and limited knowledge often make this impractical or inadvisable. Nonetheless, the selection of remedies on a first aid basis should still be according to strict homeopathic principles; the matching of symptoms to the proven remedy; the single remedy and the minimum potency necessary to trigger a healing response from the person's vital force. Many modern homeopaths, responding to the expectations of their patients, treat this way all the time. Be aware of the conditions which are beyond the scope of amateur treatment. You should always get medical assistance for critically urgent or longstanding chronic situations, though homeopathic remedies may safely relieve immediate shock while help is on the way.

The mystery of the infinitesimal dose

The homeopathic remedy can be likened to a drip of detergent in a bowl of oily water, it immediately creates a reaction across the whole surface. The remedy stimulates the healing response in a similarly dramatic way rather than by using large doses repeatedly to overwhelm or smother disease symptoms. There may well be no trace of the original source material for a remedy, once it has been diluted and succussed to become homeopathically effective. However, it is wisely said, that to value only that which is measurable, is to ignore the valuable merely because it is unmeasurable. We may know for certain that we put a cup of salt or sugar in the waters of a lake, but because water subsequently taken from it reveals no trace of the added substance, does that mean it is no longer there? No. What is at issue then is not the presence of the source substance, however unmeasurably dilute, but how it could exert any influence when diluted to such a degree.

The respectable British scientific journal, *The Lancet*, reported on 20 September 1997 that statistically quantifiable effects had been recorded when assessing well-designed trials of homeopathic remedies which were being compared with placebo treatments (imitation treatments which the patient believes to be real). In other words, these trial results were better than chance, and consistently better than occur when simply believing in the treatment. Trial results were significant to scientifically acceptable standards, even though no chemical basis for the effectiveness of the remedies could be found. *The Lancet* recommends further investigation into homeopathic effectiveness. Comparisons between homeopathic and allopathic treatments rather than comparing placebos have been problematic so far, due to the utterly opposing philosophies and methodologies which dictate any such studies are always likely to be incomparable.

What actually happens to make a remedy effective remains unclear then, but it seems homeopathy works with energy, not with the chemical properties of the substances from which it was potentized. Since it has no measurable chemical properties, it is suggested that an *energy trace* from the original substance may be affecting *energy fields* associated with the body. An analogy for this might be how two magnets of the same polarity will repel each other; just as the introduction of a homeopathically potentized substance can be observed to repel the symptoms which it matches.

The energized remedy seems to have a holographic action, because the parts of a remedy are as effective as the whole. A teaspoon of dilute remedy is not a fractional dose, but an entire one. Science is now at the point where such radical concepts can be explored experimentally. The more studies that are done, the better.

Is homeopathy safe?

Homeopathy is generally safe if its principles are adhered to; the single, well-matched remedy and the minimum potency necessary to trigger a curative response. Generally speaking the wrong remedy, if discontinued after a short period of assessment, will cause no harm whatever. Incorrectly chosen remedies usually pass through the body without effect since they find no similarity. Remedies are designed to be non-toxic after preparation by dilution and succussion, even if the original source material was poisonous. If a whole bottle-full of homeopathic tablets were taken at a single time, the remedy should do no harm. Some sceptics take this fact to be proof that homeopathic remedies cannot have any curative powers beyond those of suggestion. This is to misunderstand how the principles of similimum, potentization and the minimum dose work, by matching and influencing the body's energy patterns, rather than by altering its physical state. An accidental overdose would have the same effect as taking a single tablet, though the jolt given to the body would be far greater than necessary.

Generally, harm may occur when homeopathic principles are not well understood, or the basic tenets of homeopathy are ignored or skipped over in the amateur's haste to use homeopathic treatment. It is also possible to cause an aggravation of symptoms, as when treating chronic conditions; or to trigger an accidental proving, by continuing to give a remedy for too long, in which case the symptoms applicable to the remedy appear, rather than the restoration of health. I shall return to these topics. The homeopathic treatment of chronic conditions such as eczema and asthma should always be left to professionals, because more harm than good may be done by tinkering with the wrong remedies for problems which are already deep-seated and highly complex.

Safety was one of the motivating forces which inspired the founder of homeopathy, Samuel Hahnemann. He was sure that the harsh treatments of the conventional medicine of his day could be improved upon. He discovered potentization when experimenting to find the lowest possible, effective measure, during his clinical trials. Concerned to avoid side effects and any risks of poisoning from the toxic nature of some source materials, Hahnemann found that the remedies were safer, yet became more effective, at greater dilutions. However, he found that some remedies eventually reached a point where effectiveness remained static, yet side effects still occurred. He experimented further, making use of his chemical training and knowledge of alchemy, and found that by vigorously shaking a remedy, it remained effective at very much greater dilutions, and what is more, side effects were eliminated. Though generally safe, homeopathically prepared remedies are an influence upon the body, so their use on pregnant women, newborn babies and the very frail should always be subject to professional advice.

Homeopathy during and after pregnancy

I recommend that the amateur consult a professional homeopath when the patient is pregnant, even though many remedies are safe and beneficial at this time. Relief from many conditions such as nausea, cramping pains, threat of miscarriage and the pains of labour itself, can safely be gained from homeopathic remedies, but it is sensible to assume all medicines, even homeopathic ones, should be handled with caution at this time until you are skilled and experienced at prescribing. There is increasing concern about the risk of side effects from conventional medicines during pregnancy but with caution, most homeopathic remedies, if restricted to 6X or 12C potency, are a safe form of treatment for the pregnant or breast-feeding mother. Following the birth, the mother may safely benefit from the homeopathic treatment of conditions such as uterine cramps, cracked nipples, postnatal depression, loss of libido or haemorrhoids. Homeopathic remedies thus are an advantage at a time when allopathic medicines might be too risky, but for what to take, when, and at what potency, I still recommend professional advice to those new to homeopathy.

Combining allopathic and homeopathic remedies

A homeopathic remedy may safely be given in conjunction with allopathic medicines, but the combination can negate the effectiveness of the homeopathic remedy by antidoting it. Some homeopathic remedies are rendered ineffective or are antidoted by the taking of allopathic ones, especially steroids or antibiotics. This may become apparent when a formerly effective remedy becomes ineffectual; but if it is administered for the first time, contamination could cause a remedy to fail inexplicably. Homeopathic remedies should be taken at least 30 minutes apart from the allopathic medicine to try to avoid this invisible contamination. If it occurs, allow at least 30 minutes for the influence of the allopathic medicine to subside and give the homeopathic remedy again. So, to recap, while it does no harm to take both kinds of treatment, the homeopathic one may be rendered less effective, or even ineffective, as a result. This is **not** a recommendation to stop your conventional treatments in order to try homeopathically prepared alternatives, however. You should always take professional advice before discontinuing your conventional medicines. Some allopathic treatments can be dangerous if suddenly discontinued, and some, once started, must be taken for life. Consult your physician and a professional homeopath if you are currently receiving conventional medications which you would like to discontinue. This cannot be stressed too strongly.

Safety in acute situations

If presented with an acute emergency, such as loss of consciousness, severe injury, chest pains, headaches which affect sight, asphyxiation and other life-threatening symptoms, **call the emergency services for help first**. This is what any professional homeopath would also do. By all means then alleviate distress with well-chosen remedies and first aid if possible, but do summon help first, and mention your observations and the remedies you have given when help arrives.

The aim of this book

It is the intention of this book to teach the guiding principles by which you can select the correct remedy when faced with minor ailments and injuries. You will learn which remedies to use for first aid (symptomatic treatment) when full case taking is impossible, as well as the principles and practice of traditional homeopathy. Space limitations make it impossible to print a complete Materia Medica and Repertory which would cover all known symptom pictures, and therefore every case you might meet, but the common homeopathic first-aid treatments will be found here. The remedies in this book have been chosen for their suitability for home treatment, and providing low potencies are used, inaccurate prescribing should not exacerbate a chronic or constitutional condition. I recommend a course of basic first aid and resuscitation techniques be added to this knowledge. Equally important is knowing when to seek the advice and help of professionals such as the emergency services, allopathic doctors, and homeopathic professionals, if presented with potentially serious situations. This will be made clear where appropriate.

1 THE HISTORY AND DEVELOPMENT OF HOMEOPATHY

By similar things a disease is produced and through the application of the like it is cured.

Hippocrates

Ancient history

What is meant by homeopathy, the principles and reasons for its practice, can best be explained by the story of its discovery. So, where did it all begin? Some of the principles of what we now think of as homeopathy had been known in ancient Greece. The word homeopathy actually derives from the Greek *homoios*, meaning like and *pathos*, meaning suffering. Hippocrates, a physician in ancient Greece, identified two types of treatment. He observed that some medicines produced symptoms opposite to those caused by a disease (contraries), but that others produced the same symptoms as the disease (similars). Hippocrates concluded, therefore, that what has the power to cause suffering also has the power to heal.

Paracelsus, a notable Swiss physician and scientist of the sixteenth century, introduced many pharmaceutical remedies. He was a naturalist and a master alchemist, a forerunner of the modern chemist. Paracelsus liked to test his theories experimentally rather than rely on theories, as was the usual method in his day. He revived the idea of treatment with similars and repudiated the idea of treating with contraries. He is alleged to have said, 'Never a hot illness has been cured by something cold, nor a cold one by something hot. But it has happened that like has cured like.' With alchemical knowledge of minerals and metals, as well as knowledge of herbal remedies from his love of nature, Paracelsus was instrumental in bringing about radical changes in the medical and philosophical thinking of this time. Though controversial, his ideas eventually moved medicine away from the theoretical concept of the four humours, which had dominated notions of health and disease, medical philosophy and medical practice for centuries. We owe a debt of gratitude to Paracelsus for initiating ideas which, after his death, led to a more open-minded attitude to new ideas in medicine. The practice of clinically testing theoretical medicine was a result of his innovation, and played an essential part in the development of homeopathy.

Recent history

Homeopathy as we know it today was founded almost two hundred years ago by Samuel Christian Friedrich Hahnemann, a young doctor who was born in Saxony in 1755. A very able student, Hahnemann became disillusioned with the medical treatments he was expected to employ as a qualified, conventional physician. He was horrified by the use of harsh purgatives, high doses of poisonous mercury, and blood letting; treatments which he regarded as brutal and ineffectual, but which he was expected to use by patients and colleagues alike. Rather than continue to compromise his beliefs, in 1796 Hahnemann gave up practising as a physician, 17 years after he had qualified. To earn his living, Hahnemann then worked as a chemist, and as a translator of Greek and English medical texts; a job he had done to make ends meet when he was a medical student. Fluent in eight languages, Hahnemann had taught Greek to fellow pupils since he was aged 12. He would thus have been familiar with the ancient teachings of Hippocrates, Paracelsus and other great scholars of the past. He had always found the texts he translated more stimulating than the lectures he had heard at medical school, and, inspired by what he read, Samuel began formulating a more gentle approach to medical care.

The Law of Similars

While translating the Materia Medica of a Scottish physician, a Dr Cullen, Hahnemann became intrigued by the explanation given for the effectiveness of quinine, an extract of cinchona bark (*Cinchona calisaya*) used in the treatment of malaria. Cullen had written that he believed the effectiveness of the remedy to be due to its astringent properties, an assertion Hahnemann doubted, since he knew other astringents had no such curative effect on malaria. Following a hunch, Hahnemann began to experiment on himself, taking repeated doses of cinchona bark and noting the effects he experienced. By taking the cinchona bark himself when well, Hahnemann found he could induce the same symptoms as if he were suffering from malaria, yet the symptoms vanished when he stopped taking the remedy. This, together with what we must assume would have been his awareness of the ancient texts which recommend the treatment of like with like, was the spur Hahnemann needed to initiate further experiments upon himself, and later on willing relatives and friends. As a good scientist, Hahnemann set up his trials methodically. To avoid clouding the results, the experimental subjects had to be physically and mentally healthy, and be willing to forgo all stimulants, such as tea, coffee, alcohol or spicy foods, plus other activities which might arouse their passions! Hahnemann observed and noted their every reaction with scientific precision, calling this humane testing process *proving*. This is the term still used for the process of testing a remedy today.

Hahnemann's experimental results confirmed his hunch. As Hippocrates and Paracelsus had hinted centuries before, a medicine which produces symptoms in a healthy person can also remove those symptoms in a diseased person. By scientific experimentation, at no small risk to himself, Hahnemann could now affirm The Law of Similars, which remains at the heart of modern homeopathy; Let like be cured with like. He realized that symptoms are not, as was generally assumed, aspects of a disease. On the contrary, symptoms are indicators of the body's effort to return to health, and when a substance causes the body to produce symptoms, whatever they be, it is actually *proving* its ability to heal those symptoms, in similar disease conditions.

Hahnemann was the right man at the right time. His book, *The Organon of the Healing Art*, is still required reading for serious students of homeopathy. Many of his core ideas had been around since the time of ancient Greece, but as with other great scientific reforms, it took a visionary to bring them into a workable theory. Hahnemann had the courage to prove his theories experimentally, against the groundswell of current medical beliefs, and at the risk of his personal health and potentially lucrative career.

The Materia Medica

Hahnemann had noted that some experimental subjects experienced a greater number of reactive symptoms than others, and exhibited symptoms in varying degrees of severity. The symptoms found to be most typical or characteristic he called keynotes, while the remainder of symptoms are classified according to whether they are less often, or rarely encountered. These classifications, collected together, are the drug picture for each remedy. These meticulously recorded lists of symptom pictures gathered from Hahnemann's provings, and those produced from the observations of later homeopaths, such as Kent, remain in constant use today. They are the basis of any homeopathic Materia Medica (list of remedies), which along with a Repertory (list of symptoms), form the essential reference text books used for homeopathic prescribing. Today the categories are still laid out in the traditional order, starting with mind symptoms, then head, face, and down to the various systems of the body, the extremities and any modalities (influences noted to improve or worsen the symptoms). This traditional layout follows the homeopathic Laws of Cure which was first noted by Hering and the degree of importance attached to the symptoms. The descriptive way of recording symptoms in a Materia Medica or Repertory is called a *Rubric*. No one could effectively retain all the potential categories, combinations and modalities in memory, though the professional will become increasingly adept at recognizing the more frequently encountered ones.

Hahnemann developed a regular methodology for treatment which involved a thorough questioning of the patient, together with a physical examination and observations. He would enquire as to general health and lifestyle, moods and attitudes, present symptoms and what conditions caused them to fluctuate. Gradually Hahnemann built up a picture of this person before him and their symptoms, and believed he could recognize a similarity with a specific remedy's symptom picture. He was then able to cross-refer the patient's specific symptoms to his meticulous records of the drug pictures he had gained from the provings, and confirm which remedy was most like the symptom picture. As he had found with his personal experiments, the remedy most like the experienced symptoms was the one which alleviated them. Like did cure like. The oddest symptoms were found to be most useful in this regard. For example, a sore throat could well fit many remedies, but to discover that the throat worsened at midnight, started on the left side and followed a change in the weather, would be more helpful for identification purposes.

The infinitesimal dose

Hahnemann was not satisfied with the unpleasant side effects some patients continued to experience from the remedies he gave them, but he also had another ambition. He wanted to find a way to make safe remedies from toxic source materials, such as arsenic. He believed homeopathically prepared remedies from substances which in their natural state produce such strong symptoms would serve to alleviate symptom portraits with similar characteristics, but how to do so with poisonous materials? Hahnemann tried diluting the substances to alleviate or eliminate toxicity, side effects and aggravations. He placed some remedial source material in a solvent, usually pure alcohol or double distilled water, for a month. Next he strained off the resulting liquid, to obtain what he called a tincture, or *mother tincture*, of the original remedy. Those substances which were not soluble in alcohol or distilled water he ground up, and then dissolved into a solution, a process he called *trituration*. He then made dilutions from the mother tincture, by taking one drop of it and adding to it nine drops of pure alcohol, or distilled water. Sometimes he would add to one drop of the mother tincture 99 drops of the inert solvent or even greater dilution ratios.

Hahnemann then set about discovering whether such dilute remedies could still be clinically effective. He found from trials on himself and his human volunteers that such diluted remedies remained extremely effective; in fact more so than the original substance had been in its natural state, but that they still had limitations. He was concerned that some patients reported an aggravation, or worsening, of their symptoms. Hahnemann believed he could improve the remedies still further.

Hahnemann's next step was inspirational. At the point when he would add the single drop of mother tincture to the 99 of inert solvent (for example) he decided to shake the mixture vigorously, and bang the container on a hard surface. This seemingly odd behaviour he called *succussing*. It is possible that Hahnemann was merely using techniques he was already familiar with, from his knowledge of chemistry. In any case, succussing produced the desired effect. The remedies were now effective even beyond their already enhanced dilute limitations. He repeated this process, diluting by a fixed ratio, and each time succussing the dilute mixture. The end product of many such succussed dilutions was a solvent, which now carried no measurable trace of the substance which had formed its mother tincture, and which thus presented no risk of toxicity. The idea that a medicine could be effective without any discernable active properties, aroused controversy and disbelief among sceptics. When Hahnemann tried these diluted and apparently weakened potencies first on himself, and then on willing patients, he was amazed to discover that not only had the problem

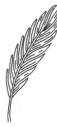

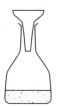

| Natural Source material | Trituration of non-soluble source material | Soluble/ triturated material steeped in dilution of alcohol or pure water | Mother tincture | Potentized remedy (mother tincture further diluted and succussed to the desired potency) |

Figure 3   Dilution, trituration and succussion

of side effects, aggravations and toxicity which he had sought to address been resolved, but that these diluted remedies worked much faster, and more effectively, than their supposedly stronger precursors, and were in fact more potent. Even a normally toxic substance, if diluted, succussed and potentized in this way, could be made into a safe and effective remedy.

Hahnemann continued to test the remedies in these smaller doses, and an ever more diluted form, to see if they would remain effective. They did. Another basic tenet of homeopathic treatment had been discovered; the principle of the minimum dose. Hahnemann had confirmed, to his own satisfaction, that symptoms, rather than being evidence of the presence of a disease, were actually evidence of a body's attempt to heal itself, by reacting to threat or stress. Hahnemann believed the remedies were triggering what he called the vital force, or natural curative response of the individual, by their being similar to the reactions resulting from the original agent of stress. Now Hahnemann could begin to practise medicine as he had wanted to when young, by the gentlest means possible, rather than by using the brutal methods of current orthodoxy. As a result of continued experimentation by followers of Hahnemann, homeopathic treatments are nowadays available in even greater dilutions, and in various forms; as pills, phials, potions, lotions, creams, wafers, and so on, according to the sensitivities of the patient and the suitability of administration.

Constitutional types, miasms and psora

Hahnemann's work was still not yet complete. He began to realize that some people expressed predictable groups of symptoms, which could be described as reflecting their constitutional type. Chronic illness involves repetitive and unpredictable cycles of health and disease. Hahnemann noted an overall downward spiral in the chronic disease pattern. He noted these patients' health histories. There were periods when the person's vital force had succumbed to stress, giving rise to a familiar symptom picture, which then alternated with periods of health, when the vital force repelled dis-ease. Some patients showed this taint, or predisposition to a recognizable symptom portrait, which Hahnemann called a *miasm*. It seemed to him that some chronic conditions, or miasms, were a continuing response to a past exposure to particular micro-organisms. He called such influences *psora*. Hahnemann was now able to help patients in a way that had been impossible with the conventional treatments of his day. He could select the remedy which would boost the patient's own natural will to health, and by stimulating healthy vitality, enable the person to shrug off stress, and even prevent illness developing.

The treatment of miasms, psora and some other chronic prescribing, is not suitable for the inexperienced homeopath, and such an advanced level of homeopathic competence is well beyond the limited scope of this book. It takes great skill and experience to assess these longstanding symptom patterns successfully, and to treat the levels of reactive symptoms they have produced delicately. Therefore, this sort of constitutional prescribing should be left strictly to the professional homeopath. However, it is impossible to treat homeopathically, at even a limited level, without some awareness of the constitutional principles upon which the remedy descriptions are based. For this reason, and for the serious student of homeopathy, I shall briefly and simply explain what is meant by the term constitutional type.

We all know of the person who works and plays hard, eats a poor diet, drinks too much alcohol and smokes habitually yet is never ill, while his or her careful and abstemious neighbour seems to become unwell whenever the wind changes direction. The difference lies with their genetically inherited constitutions. Though the first character may take health for granted, as well he or she may, continued stress may eventually exact a price. Similarly the less fortunate neighbour may marshall his or her resources to best effect, and remain generally well. Then there is the example of the nurse who always becomes ill with headaches, vomiting and fever when exposed to infections, whereas a colleague remains unaffected by exposure to the same risk factors. The first nurse would seem to have an inherent weakness to bacterial infections, which the second nurse plainly does not. A third nurse exposed to the same level of risk might manifest completely different symptoms of dis-ease to the first, and a fourth nurse yet another variation, as a habitual response to bacterial exposure. Constitutional types reveal a predisposition to suffer specific groups of symptoms. It is the recognition of such symptom portraits that guides the classical homeopath to the remedy which in the healthy person produces a matching symptom picture. Thus we can speak of the Euphrasia type, or the Gelsemium type, and though each person will manifest common features too, it is by recognizing the characteristic and distinguishing features of a remedy that the patient may be constitutionally prescribed.

Professionally trained homeopaths today can prescribe specifically for the constitutional type. They can anticipate susceptibilities and give preventative care, rather than await the breakdown of the body's defenses. Taking a remedy before you are feeling sick is called homeoprophylaxis, or immunization by homeopathy. Such prescribing aims to build up the patient's innate vital force and response to dis-ease, given each patient's unique susceptibility.

The cholera outbreak

In 1831 Hahnemann published papers on the homeopathic treatment of cholera symptoms, a dis-ease then spreading through Europe at an alarming rate. In the areas where his suggested treatments for medication and hygiene were employed, the cure rate was impressive. Mortality rates from cholera under homeopathic treatment varied between 2.4 and 21.1 per cent, whereas 50 per cent or more had died when given conventional treatments. Similar successes were reported from homeopathic treatment during other epidemics, including meningitis, yellow fever and scarlet fever outbreaks.

Constantine Hering

Hahnemann died in 1843 at the age of 88. His published work remains in print and is still in daily use worldwide. Hahnemann's work has been admired and extended by later homeopaths. Constantine Hering (1800–1880) was one such early convert. He studied conventional medicine at Leipzig and originally shared the medical faculty's low opinion of homeopathy. Asked to research and write a paper to disprove Hahnemann's work he was pleased to do so, but the more Hering learned of homeopathy, the more impressed he became, especially after he had a personal encounter with its effectiveness. He had a badly infected hand which was not responding to conventional treatment, and which as a result was threatened with amputation. In desperation he tried homeopathy, and cured the infection. Unable to continue with this critical paper in the face of such personal proof, he abandoned it and changed to another university where he might learn more about homeopathy, without the hostility he knew he would encounter at Leipzig. Hering travelled widely and tested, or proved, many remedies during the rest of his life, using materials he encountered on his travels. He recorded his results, aided by his wife, and added a great deal to the body of homeopathic knowledge. Hering eventually moved to America and founded a highly influential training college, and a hospital which treated many thousands of patients.

Hering's Laws of Cure

Hering remains famous for having observed and described the natural progression of healing, which is known as Hering's Laws of Cure. This states that symptoms disappear in the reverse order of their appearance, and also in a specific sequence. Symptoms affecting upper areas of the body clear before those affecting lower areas, for example, brain symptoms clear before a knee problem; symptoms clear from the inside before the outside, i.e. a stomach problem, being deeper in the system, will clear before an ankle problem; and symptoms clear from more vital organs before less vital organs, i.e. from the heart before the stomach. Therefore during homeopathic treatment, old symptoms may return as they are worked out of the system, which may seem like a relapse if the patient has not been warned to expect this.

Hering also greatly extended Hahnemann's work on miasms, but not without controversy. In proving substances based on the products of dis-ease, such as phlegm or sputum, some say he strayed from the principle of treating like with like. In using remedies such as these, Hering was accused of treating like with the same, a subtle difference. Treating with extracts of the effects of dis-ease is more like the principles of immunization than of

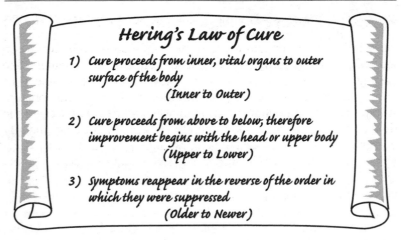

Hering's Law of Cure

1) *Cure proceeds from inner, vital organs to outer surface of the body*
   (Inner to Outer)

2) *Cure proceeds from above to below, therefore improvement begins with the head or upper body*
   (Upper to Lower)

3) *Symptoms reappear in the reverse of the order in which they were suppressed*
   (Older to Newer)

Figure 4   The Laws of Cure

homeopathy. It is a subtle distinction. Hahnemann's methodology involves stimulation of the body's own healing (vital) force by matching like symptoms. Samuel Hahnemann had stated it is by introducing stronger symptoms to those being suffered that the whole disease is eradicated.

James Tyler Kent (1849–1916)

James Kent, born in the United States of America, became a convert when he witnessed the homeopathic cure of his wife. He researched and experimented with provings and potencies, and added much to modern knowledge. However, he has always been somewhat controversial among fellow homeopaths for his habit of using higher potencies than those Hahnemann had advocated, a practice which seems to deviate from the principle of the infinitesimal dose. Kent's work remains controversial and extremely influential today. During his career he published many homeopathic text books. These include an improved Homeopathic Materia Medica with more easily recognized descriptions; an extremely helpful Repertory of the homeopathic Materia Medica; and a Philosophy of Homeopathy. These are still standard texts used by modern homeopaths every day.

Frederick Hervey Foster Quin (1799–1879)

Quin did much to encourage the use of homeopathy in Britain in the 1830s. He had formerly met and studied with Hahnemann. Like Hering and Kent, he personally experienced the efficacy of homeopathy. In his case he was cured of cholera by Hahnemann, who prescribed Camphor for his symptom picture. Quin treated the rich and famous in London society, where he became socially powerful. His well-placed connections proved to be beneficial when the House of Lords later attempted to suppress homeopathy. Quin founded the London Homeopathic Hospital in 1849 (later to be called the Royal London Homeopathic Hospital, when it received Royal patronage).

Homeopathy today

Combination remedies

The homeopathy practised by Hahnemann has been developed and extended, though not without controversy. Remedy combining is practised today in some parts of the world, notably France and Germany, and to some extent in Britain and the United States. Companies market combinations of remedies, all of which are believed to operate on a similar group of symptoms, such as in cases of depression, or the menopause. The assumption is that the wrong remedies will have no effect while the right remedy, hopefully among those combined, will trigger the curative reaction. Combining remedies in this way paves the way for marketing according to generalized pathological symptoms, and for greater use of remedies without the need or benefit of a professional homeopath. There is no need for individual case-taking, which saves on the time and expertise needed to select the single, individualized remedy accurately. This form of prescribing is contrary to Hahnemann's classical methodology because the substances were proved singly, so their effects when taken in combination are untested. *'In no case is it necessary and therefore not permissible to administer to a patient more than one single, simple medicinal substance at one time.'* (Organon § 273). Hahnemann defined what he meant by simple remedies quite precisely so combination treatments break with tradition. However, combination remedies though inimical to classical principles, have brought awareness of homeopathy, in name at least, to a wider public. Perhaps combinations of remedies will be proved one day, and homeopathic knowledge will be expanded to include them, but meanwhile, the single remedy and the lowest possible potency remains classical practice.

Remedy affinities

Remedy affinities are another matter. It has long been noted that certain remedies, given one after the other, match the movement of disease symptoms beneficially and complement each other well, or are at least known to have an affinity of action. Also known are inimicals, the relationships which do not happily follow on from each other. These known remedy relationships are a valuable part of the treatment for chronic conditions which should only be attempted by the professionally trained homeopath. Remedy relationships do adhere to classical principles because each is given singly and time is allowed for its effect. These relationships are tried and tested and are quoted in the repertories accompanying professional Materia Medica, along with the suggested duration of each remedy before moving to the next.

Sarcodes, Nosodes and Imponderabilia

Since Hahnemann's day, Sarcodes, Nosodes and Imponderabilia have been added to the lists of source materials subjected to rigorous proving. Sarcodes are homeopathically prepared from animal secretions such as dog's milk, and animal tissue such as thyroid extract, which will have been taken from the thyroid gland of a young calf or sheep. Nosodes are prepared from morbid secretations or tissues, which may be of human origin. Bacillinum for example, is the macerated tissue of a tuberculous lung, while Vaccininum is prepared from vaccine material. Even more surprising sources perhaps, are the aptly called Imponderabilia. These include exposure to X-ray, electricity, magnetic forces, and so on. Though mentioned because they are a part of the professional homeopath's pharmacy, the use of Nosodes, Sarcodes and Imponderabilia are beyond the prescribing scope of this book.

Worldwide homeopathy

Homeopathy is growing in popularity worldwide but is especially accepted as an alternative treatment to allopathy in Germany, France, Great Britain and India. Homeopathy has been practised in the United States for nearly two hundred years, and although today it is not widely accepted as a reputable alternative to conventional medicine, that picture is changing. Many American orthodox practitioners have expressed an interest in learning more about homeopathy. In Greece, George Vithoulkas has greatly extended the scope of homeopathy, and has published many important works, trained many colleagues, and treated many patients in recent years. In Britain today homeopathy is increasingly accepted as a respectable example of several alternatives to conventional treatment. Professional homeopaths are regulated and registered, and some conventional doctors have also trained in homeopathic principles. There are also several homeopathic hospitals in Great Britain.

2 | HOMEOPATHY ON TRIAL

A history of resistance

Ever since Hahnemann first practised homeopathy, its principles have been attacked by various members of the orthodox medical profession. Apothecaries objected to the fact that Hahnemann prepared his own medicines and in 1820 brought a legal injunction against him in an attempt to forbid him doing so. If all doctors prepared their own medicines it could threaten pharmacists' livelihoods.

American medical orthodoxy grew to be especially critical of homeopathy. The expansion of conventional medicine early in the twentieth century meant allopathic specialists could command high incomes commensurate with valuable skills. Many American homeopaths who had provided satisfactory healthcare to generations of the same families now noticed a fall in their income. It seems that driven by financial necessity more and more of them switched to allopathic treatments for a higher income per hour of work. Those homeopaths who chose to stay with their discipline had to compete for the care of patients and a livelihood with an increasingly large number of allopaths. It is suspected in some quarters that opposition to homeopathy today is still not solely predicated on issues of disease and cure. Allopathic medical practitioners still enjoy a lucrative professional status where healthcare is not free and this might be lessened if homeopathy become popular. In Great Britain, for example, where healthcare is free and state funded unless the patient elects otherwise, competition for income scarcely arises. Homeopathy in Britain is increasingly accepted as a legitimate alternative by conventional medical practitioners who may even refer patients on for treatment by a homeopath, or to a homeopathic hospital, if the patient requests it or a chronic condition suggests it. Where competition for patient income exists, homeopathy meets powerful opposition from orthodoxy.

Whatever the reason, historically there has been great resistance to homeopathy in the United States of America, despite its early success there. (The American Institute of Homeopathy was founded in 1844, two years before the founding of the orthodox American Medical Association (AMA).) Considerable opposition and hostility remains despite the fact that in America, homeopathic practitioners can only legally practise after having first completed their training in conventional medicine. These stalwart homeopaths deem it worthwhile to spend the extra time, effort and expense necessary to become accredited homeopaths, to practise what they believe in. However, perhaps negative reactions to homeopathy in America are about to change. A survey conducted by researchers at the University of Maryland of primary care physicians (members of the AMA) revealed that 49 per cent of them would be interested to train in homeopathy (*British Homeopathic Journal*, July, 1997). The same researchers surveyed Maryland family practice doctors, and discovered that 69 per cent would be interested in homeopathic training (*Journal of the American Board of Family Practice*, 1995, 8).

The accusations

The notion that greatly diluted and succussed substances could be effective is the target for most criticism levelled at homeopathy. If a substance is so dilute that no trace of the original, active property can be detected in the solution, how can it possibly be claimed to effect a cure? It defies the logic of observable cause and effect, and affronts those who require a reasonable explanation before they will accept practical evidence of success. Detractors seeking to explain the inexplicable have accused patients of merely responding with a placebo effect, of delusional wishful thinking, to explain away successful cures.

Accusations rebuffed

Accusations of delusional wishful thinking seem inappropriate when levelled at infants or animals, and can hardly be levelled at plants, yet when tested, all these have shown positive reactions to homeopathic treatments which were statistically better than chance. Such subjects were plainly in complete ignorance of scientific contention or debate, and had no comprehension of the difference between a homeopathic and an allopathic treatment. The reactions measured were of the effects of application(s) of homeopathic remedy(ies) under scientifically rigorous conditions (without comparison to allopathic medicines or placebos). A trial of homeopathic remedies on breeding pigs was completed in 1984. Results showed a reduction of 10 per cent in their rate of stillbirths as compared to the control group not so treated, and many similar studies in France have given results favourable to homeopathy.

The original provings of the remedies by Hahnemann and his followers have also been attacked as being unreliable for using subjective, potentially biased accounts; and for not having been subject to strict trial conditions. To test such assertions many remedies have been proved again in America, under modern rigorous conditions. The test subjects did not know what remedy they were proving, and in the re-proving of Belladonna, did not even know if they were given a placebo, yet the resulting symptom pictures matched the traditional remedy portraits exactly. It will be interesting if the scientific will currently expended on trying to disprove homeopathic principles is ever spent on understanding how and why it does work.

Homeopathy *vs.* placebos on trial

A small (24 patients) clinical trial recently evaluated homeopathic medicine for the treatment of asthma. Researchers at the University of Glasgow used conventional allergy testing to discover which substances these asthma patients were most allergic to, then the subjects were randomized into treatment and placebo groups. Those patients chosen for treatment were given the 30C potency of the substance to which they were most allergic and were assessed by homeopathic and conventional physicians. Eighty-two per cent of the patients given a homeopathic medicine improved, compared to 38 per cent of patients given a placebo. Asked if they felt the patient received the homeopathic medicine or the placebo, both the patients and the doctors tended to guess correctly.

The respected medical publication, *The Lancet*, in its 20 September, 1997 (350/9081) edition, reported a meta-analysis of 89 blinded, randomized, placebo-controlled clinical trials (terms denoting scientifically rigorous methodology). The selected trials met strict criteria: Sample size, since drop-outs might have influenced results by affecting sample size and thereby the predetermined selection criteria; the use of control groups (people included in a study who are not given any medication, for comparative purposes); and whether the trials were blind, or double blind, to avoid unwitting or deliberate influence from the administrators of the trials. (In a blind trial the administrator knows who receives the medication and who the placebo, but the volunteer taking the medication does not; in a double blind trial neither administrator nor volunteer knows who has received the medicine and who received the placebo, due to the way the trial is set up. Double blind trials are regarded as more scientific as they rule out the possibility of the experimenter knowingly, or unconsciously, exerting influence with their own bias.) When the 89 selected trials were pooled together, results showed that homeopathic medicines had a 2.45 times greater effect than placebos. *The Lancet* suggests that since the results defy the statistical probability of chance, homeopathy at least deserves more research.

Unfair comparisons

There is a basic problem when comparing allopathic and homeopathic medicines in any trial, because the core beliefs which underpin each method are so opposed. To provide the conditions which would enable a reasonable trial of either type of medicine, involves compromising the conditions required for testing the other. This is true whether the trial is set up to meet allopathic or homeopathic treatment conditions. The allopathic trial selects a number of volunteers who are deemed to suffer from the same, identifiable condition for whom the same drug or treatment is prescribed. There is a tacitly assumed state of health compared with which disease can be identified, though what does constitute a healthy person is not defined.

Allopathic test volunteers are selected for similarity of symptoms and for suffering a named pathology (disease). In contrast, a homeopathic trial treats each volunteer as unique and therefore seeks out symptom differences, rather than common symptoms. From the identifiable differences found in each homeopathic volunteer, many different remedies may be selected, each tailored to the symptoms of the individual. There would be no universal remedy identified as a treatment for a common pathological condition, according to classical homeopathy. There are as many common colds as the people who experience them. Trials have also neglected to address differences in the normal prescribing method of each discipline. Homeopathic patients are usually monitored for alterations in their symptoms, with changes made to the remedy prescribed if appropriate; whereas the allopathic trials are set up to administer the same drug throughout the trial. The variability which is an essential element of homeopathic prescribing makes trial comparisons with allopathic prescribing very difficult. Just what homeopathic remedy did do what?

There is another barrier to sensible comparisons. In the homeopathic trials conducted so far the volunteers have continued to take their allopathic medicines while trialling the homeopathic ones. Because the volunteers are real patients it was deemed unethical to withdraw their conventional medicines for the purposes of a trial, especially as under test conditions some receive only placebo treatment. The problem is that many allopathic medicines neutralize or contaminate homeopathic remedies, though the reverse is not the case. This creates a one-way handicap which disadvantages homeopathy. For all these reasons, the trials which have been assessed have not made meaningful comparisons easy. That nonetheless there are proven, independently verified, statistically significant results which favour homeopathy is thus all the more remarkable. Even with unfavourable test parameters, homeopathic treatments have sometimes outclassed their equivalent allopathic treatments in trials. This is especially true of patients exhibiting chronic symptoms, such as the pathology known as asthma or eczema, who showed no improvement from allopathic treatment but showed marked improvement when given the individually appropriate homeopathic remedy. Homeopaths are pleased to have scientific confirmation of what they know from practical experience.

In life, rather than trials, so long as allopathy remains the first choice treatment for most people, homeopaths are mainly consulted for worst-case conditions, which of their nature may be harder to treat. Homeopaths are also often consulted only after allopathic treatments have proved disappointing. This presents other difficulties for the homeopath, who must recognize which symptoms have been caused by taking the allopathic medicines, and which pertain to the original complaint. This adds an unfair handicap if making comparisons with allopathy, which is unaffected by prior homeopathic prescribing. That homeopathy still succeeds in treating patients so startlingly well despite such handicaps is a further testament to its efficacy.

It is possible that recent developments in physics may lead to scientific explanations for what is presently inexplicable; how homeopathic remedies induce a cure when no active trace of the original substance remains. Up to now the active presence within the remedy could only be inferred, like the ripples from a pebble thrown into a pond, by the ripples or results it produced. There is speculation that the electromagnetic field of the patient's body is subtly affected by the remedy. This theory suggests the remedy carries an electromagnetic trace of the core substance from which it originated, as a result of succussion (vigorous shaking) and dilution. This may then act as a catalyst on the body to trigger the healing reaction, or alternatively may have a more direct affect on the body's own electromagnetic field, harmonically fine-tuning it towards equilibrium, by the influence of its presence.

It is common pharmacological knowledge that while a large amount of poison can kill and a lesser amount can maim, a tiny amount can simply stimulate. With this understanding, allopathic doctors frequently prescribe anticoagulants to discourage blood clotting in human patients at risk of thromboses. This medicine is prescribed in doses small enough to stimulate blood flow, when larger does would be fatal, since the same substance in a stronger concentration induces haemorrhages. Samuel Hahnemann, founder of homeopathy, had discovered that the greater the number of dilutions and succussions, the greater the potency of the remedy. Less is more. Since a potentized remedy triggers the body's own healing response, it is not necessary to flood the body with large doses, as if illness could be supplanted or drowned by large volumes of the remedy. Large applications of the original substance from which a remedy is homeopathically prepared might be ineffectual, harmful or even deadly, but the potentized remedy, prepared from the same core substance, harmlessly triggers a cure. The homeopath will use only the minimum dose needed to trigger a cure.

That the minimum dose works should not be in doubt when one considers that animals and even plants so treated cannot know a homeopathic pill from an allopathic one, unlike more suggestible humans, yet the influence of a homeopathic remedy is clearly obvious and repeatable under scientific conditions. Until explanations are forthcoming which meet with the criteria of science, or until science expands its criteria of what science is, we must rely on observation and experience only. Orthodoxy has defined as scientific only that which matches the methodology of orthodoxy. By such a circular, tautological system of definition, only those processes which match orthodox methods and expectations can be called scientific. In other words, alternative philosophies and methodologies cannot possibly be scientific, when to be scientific is to be orthodox, by definition. The system with the most adherents defines the criteria for all. Like a game of noughts and crosses, or tic tac toe, whoever calls first will win such an argument.

3 | WHAT DOES HOMEOPATHIC TREATMENT INVOLVE?

The physician's highest and only calling is to restore health to the sick, which is called healing.

Samuel Hahnemann: *The Organon of the Healing Art*

Individual treatment

All homeopathy involves the treatment of an individual patient, a person whose natural state of health has become unbalanced. A potentized and diluted agent known to produce similar symptoms in a healthy person to those now causing problems, is given to the patient; the treatment of like with like. The effect of this is to trigger the person's own healing response which will restore equilibrium. Homeopathic remedies are usually administered orally, and are only tested on human volunteers. Though energized, they are so diluted that their effect on the body and its immune system is gentle. Sceptics doubt how anything so dilute can produce these effects.

Conventional medicine involves treatment by means of opposites, so a patient who exhibits fever symptoms would be prescribed medicine which should reduce fever. Homeopaths regard treatment with opposites as suppressive and unhelpful, since the short-term removal of external symptoms merely encourages disease to penetrate to deeper levels of the body, where it will be more dangerous and difficult to treat in the long term. Removing symptoms negates the body's attempt to restore health, and obscures the basis of the original dis-ease condition. The classical homeopath, knowing which remedies will induce a fever in a healthy person, would prescribe a minimum potency of the similimum which most nearly matches the whole symptom picture of the individual, (having assessed changes from the norm in the physical, mental and emotional realms and any causal situations). The similimum is intended to trigger the body's innate defence in reaction to the stimulus. The homeopathic method encourages the patient to self-healing, rather than introduce influence designed to block, mask or counteract symptoms. Symptoms appear before deterioration occurs deeper in the body, so if heeded, they can be an accurate means of preventing more harmful structural damage.

The stages of cure

According to Hering, dis-ease passes from an acute phase through ever-deepening stages to become a chronic condition as symptoms are suppressed. The symptoms which had appeared first, however long ago, will be the last to re-emerge as the cure progresses in a reversal of this suppression. The greatest threat to well being will be resolved before lesser threats, so the threat to the deepest and most critical organs will clear first. To refresh your memory, Hering's Laws of Cure stated:

1 Cure progresses from inner organs outwards towards the surface of the body.
2 Cure proceeds from above to below, so the first improvement will be evident in the head or upper body.
3 Previously suppressed symptoms will reappear in reverse of the order in which they were suppressed.

The re-emergence of previously troublesome symptoms may suggest one is succumbing again to previously cured problems, but their appearance is a welcome sign of improvement to the homeopath. In addition, symptoms affecting the upper body will clear before those affecting the lower body and those affecting the inner body before the outer. Hering also knew that since only one illness affects a person at any time, though its symptom manifestations may be varied and may change over time, mental illness should not to be regarded as a separate or different category of disease. It is evidence of an illness which once had its acute origins elsewhere in the body but which eventually progressed to affect this vital organ inside the top of the body. Hering formulated the Laws of Cure which remains a basic tenet of homeopathy today:

Healing proceeds from within to without, from above to below, and from vital organs to less vital organs; and all in the reverse of the order in which symptoms appeared. It is a rule in homeopathy that any symptoms affecting the skin, as an outer and less vital organ, should not be suppressed. To do so would merely drive illness inwards and cause it to manifest more seriously elsewhere at a later time. Skin conditions such as eczema should therefore be left to the professional to treat.

Aggravations, from better to worse

The well-chosen similimum may have unseated a deeply submerged symptom. As a result, long forgotten symptoms may re-emerge as the body's vital force gradually restores equilibrium, sometimes to the horror of the patient. These apparently new symptoms should not be prescribed for. They should appear only fleetingly during a progression towards health. To treat them would merely suppress them again. The homeopath, who knows Hering's law states symptoms will reappear in the reverse order to their suppression, sees evidence of the deepest symptoms returning as a good sign, so long as they are part of a progression towards more surface symptoms. In practice, this may mean that the inner organs, such as the heart, liver or lungs will be the first to show a reaction to the given remedy, and the less critical symptoms, often evident on the surface, such as those affecting the skin, sleep patterns or bowel habits, will disappear last. If the patient has forgotten the progression of the symptoms when they were first experienced and suppressed, as may be the case with longstanding illness, what to the homeopath is a welcome sign of the progress towards cure may seem an alarming relapse.

How to select the single remedy?

Just as the child has to learn to discriminate from the sea of faces it encounters, so the homeopath must seek out the nuances which define and differentiate a remedy picture, not the symptoms which commonly unite sufferers of a disease, as is the practice with allopathic diagnoses. At first it may seem daunting to learn so many peculiar symptoms but no one relies on memory for all the indicators of a remedy picture; this is why we have the *Materia Medica* and *Repertory*. It is perfectly normal for a homeopath to be surrounded with huge battered text books and to refer to them when actually taking the case history. Homeopathy involves the precise matching of symptom pictures, not the following of hunches.

Labelling anomalies in the USA

The multiplicity of symptoms has created a problem when purchasing a remedy in the USA. According to FDA rules, the packaging of a homeopathic remedy must be identified by means of a single keynote symptom. The label is thus a single generalization taken from the long list of possible descriptive symptoms in the Materia Medica, which all apply to the same remedy. This can confuse any purchaser of a homeopathic remedy who is unaware of this rule. This artificial specificity may suggest that this is not the remedy one needs because it seems to bear no relation to the symptoms one wanted to treat. Homeopathic remedies cannot be labelled appropriately with a single identifier, yet they must be, since this is the law. You should bear this anomaly in mind if purchasing a homeopathic remedy in the USA.

Constitutional homeopathy

Chronic and constitutional treatments require skills and experience beyond the scope of this book and its Materia Medica. However, some understanding of the philosophy of constitutional treatment may serve to emphasize why certain elements are also important, even when assessing acute remedies. One person may take great care of his or her health and hygiene yet is prone to repetitive bouts of illness, while another who takes no care at all, and even seems to abuse his or her body, appears to keep perfect health. The difference lies in their constitutional natures. This diversity of constitutional susceptibilities allows healthcare workers to treat others' illnesses without necessarily succumbing themselves. Vulnerability to dis-ease is thus a combination of inheritance and present stress, be that emotional, mental, physical or environmental. We know that not everyone exposed to an infectious disease becomes ill with it. Those who do become ill, do so because they had a pre-existing susceptibility, perhaps combined with some short-term stress factors which together made them more vulnerable to infectious attack on this occasion. Those not affected, though their exposure was equally great, evidently had a stronger, presently unstressed consitution, and perhaps different innate susceptibilities. Modern urban living creates a great deal of stress. Those who do not recognize signs of their weakened resistance become ill repeatedly with minor conditions. The reckless person, even if possessed of a strong constitution, will be called to account by his or her body one day if the advantage is continually squandered. Even an inherited resistance to harmful environmental factors cannot resist a continual onslaught without breaking down. In contrast, the cautious person will recognize a constitutional weakness and susceptibility to external influences, and act to remedy the situation. This could involve recognizing signs of stress and taking avoiding action; getting enough sleep, exercise and a healthy diet. In addition, the person aware of his or her susceptibility to frequent illness may visit a professional homeopath to assess the appropriate constitutional remedy with which to strengthen his or her vital force. Constitutional homeopathy treats the whole person by boosting the vital force, the natural immunity to disease, and so

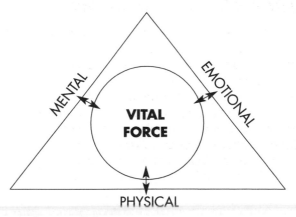

Figure 5   The vital force

counteracts the disadvantages of inheritance and early life. A strengthened constitution can better withstand the stresses which we all become exposed to at one time or another. Constitutional prescribing can respond to susceptibilities rather than wait for a dis-ease reaction to stress. The methodology remains valid when selecting any remedy, though is more extensive than may be practical for first-aid situations.

4 | PHARMACY AND POTENCY

Pharmacy describes the preparation necessary to elicit the mother tincture, the basis of a remedy, from the source material. If the basic substance is soluble it is steeped in pure alcohol or double distilled water. Non-soluble raw materials are first triturated (ground with a mortar and pestle) before being diluted in alcohol or distilled water in a similar way. After a predetermined time, the mixture is strained keeping only the alcohol or distilled water which has been affected by the recent presence of the substance. Scientific analysis at this stage would probably find traces of the basic material in the alcohol or distilled water mixture. The resulting tincture is an effective remedy, though not as powerful as it becomes after potentization. Unlike allopathic medicines which become less effective when diluted, the more dilute a homeopathic remedy, the more powerful its curative properties become, especially if potentized. The mother tincture, or tincture as the distilled water or alcohol mixture is properly called, is now diluted further, according to the pharmacist's requirements.

The decimal scale of dilution

The decimal scale involves adding one drop of mother tincture to nine drops of dilutant, the resulting dilution usually described as 1X (or 1D, or simply 1). Diluting in this way in a ratio of one drop to nine drops, each time starting with a drop of the previously diluted tincture, the modern pharmacist produces dilutions of 2X, 3X, up to 6X, 30X, and so on. (So 2X is produced by adding one drop of tincture to nine drops of dilutant, then a single drop taken from the succussed result is added to a further nine drops of dilutant.) The greater the number of dilutions, the more powerful the remedy. Less is more as regards traces of the original source material, so a 6X remedy consists of 1 part mother tincture in 1,000,000 parts alcohol/water. Once potencies are diluted to 30X and above, no molecules of the mother tincture remain.

The centesimal scale of dilution

The centesimal scale of dilution produces even more powerful remedies due to the increased amount of dilution and number of succussions. To produce dilutions in the centesimal scale the pharmacist adds one drop of mother tincture to 99 drops of dilutant, continuing in increments of one to hundred, as its name suggests. These are described as 1C, 2C, up to 200C or more. Strengths above 30C should not be administered by the amateur, as by proving they could introduce the symptoms with which they are associated, even when not the remedy for the present condition. Higher potencies still are produced purely for expert use. These may be as great as 5M (diluted five thousand times) or even CM (a hundred thousand dilutions). These higher potencies are usually designated just by number, 100, 200, 100,000, and so on, sometimes written as 100C, 200C, CM, for example.

Succussion

When Hahnemann proved the original remedies he found there was a limit to their effectiveness by dilution. Eventually a point was reached where no reaction occurred in the volunteer, and therefore no curative response could be expected if it were given to a sick person. We assume Hahnemann now utilized his experience as a translator of alchemical and chemical treatises because he decided to shake the diluted remedy vigorously, and found by doing so its effectiveness was greatly enhanced. What is more, the toxic aggravations and reactions he had been trying to limit, by diluting the source material, diminished or disappeared altogether. This was a breakthrough. Vigorous shaking and tapping of the container holding the dilute remedy, called succussion (vibration), is now standard practice for potentizing a remedy in whatever dilution. The action of shaking the dilute substance dynamically potentizes its energy so the risk of toxic side effects is minimized and the remedy made more powerful. The greater the number of dilutions and potentizations, the stronger the remedy. Potentization describes how the mother tincture is rendered more homeopathically effective by the process of succussion, and potency is the strength of the resulting remedy. Once the process of dilution and succussion has been completed the number of times necessary for the intended potency, a few drops are added to an inert carrier, typically saccharum lactose tablets or pillules (sac lac), taken orally.

It is another axiom of homeopathy that a remedy should be taken in the minimum dose possible to initiate the curative response. (Dose equates to potency, since each application of a remedy is entire and should not be thought of as acting on an accumulative basis, as would be the case with some allopathic medicines.) How much constitutes a minimum dose will vary according to the nature of the complaint and the severity of the symptoms. This is important because if more than the minimum necessary dose is taken, it can cause a proving rather than a cure. The capability of the minimum dose to trigger a healing response will have been lost and replaced with an accidental proving of the remedy, with the result that new symptoms have been introduced. What this means in practice is the accidental production of the telltale symptoms associated with the remedy, some of which were not part of the original problem but which will now also require treatment. If this occurs it is advisable to seek professional help to untangle the complication of symptoms and their causes.

5 | PRACTICALITIES: FIRST AID AND ACUTE TREATMENT

First aid treatment

The methods of assessment and prescribing suitable for acute treatment or first aid will of necessity differ from your treatment of non-emergency acute situations. With no time or opportunity to take a lengthy case history, you need to make a symptomatic choice from the remedies known to relieve the stress of trauma. That said, the remedy you select will still follow homeopathic principles in being the most suitable for the symptoms you are presented with, as well as your knowledge of what has just occurred. In addition, you will treat only as long as it takes to see a marked improvement, and no longer. Once the patient is comfortable you may have time to take the case properly and select the remedy which fits his or her wider symptom picture. So, in an emergency, base your selection on the remedy picture which as far as possible matches the most urgent symptoms. Do not worry if your case does not match all the possible features of a stated remedy picture, though it should match the defining characteristics.

Potencies for first aid

You will recall that potentization is the energizing preparation of a mother tincture to render it more homeopathically effective. This is done by the process of succussion (repeated dilution and vibration). Potency is the strength of the resulting remedy. Low potencies such as 6X, 9X, 12X, and 30X; or 6C, 12C and 30C are the only strengths advisable for amateur use, though there are much greater potencies available to the professionally trained homeopath. When you see homeopathic remedies described as 6X they are at a low potency. The higher the X or C factor, the greater the number of times the mother tincture was diluted and succussed and consequently, the stronger the remedy. As a generalization, use lower potencies when the presenting condition is largely physical in nature, and higher potencies, which penetrate deeper, when the presenting symptoms are predominantly emotional or mental in nature.

Base the potency you give for first aid on the severity and urgency of the symptoms; 30C in a single dose if symptoms are severe; alternatively 6C or 12C with repeated doses as necessary. Prescribing potencies and doses according to degrees of severity are described at length in the section on acute treatment, but basically, the greater the pain, the higher the potency and the sooner the repetition if symptoms relapse. If necessary, adjust the dose and frequency to the potency of remedy available, giving longer between repeats if you have only a stronger potency than is recommended, and repeating more frequently if the reverse.

Always be guided by observation of the patient. Stop as soon as improvement is noted and extend the period before treating again. Stop altogether when a definite curative response is noted, such as a healthy sleep or feeling of well being. Be alert to the possibility of new symptoms which will require a different remedy, bearing in mind the laws of cure and the possibility of aggravating an earlier condition; and if no response occurs after a reasonable time, reconsider your choice of remedy.

First aid frequency and dose

Give an initial dose, repeat until improvement is noted, then pause and consider the following options:

- If symptoms return, repeat this cycle three to six times until improvement is well established.
- If marked improvement is evident, stop all treatment. Repeat only if the same symptoms later return. Observe for laws of cure.
- If no improvement occurs, try a different remedy or if different symptoms appear which suggest aggravation, consult a professional.
- If symptoms become alarming, continue unabated, or get worse, call for professional help.

The remedies for symptomatic first aid

Bites, stings: Apis Mel; Led; Hyp; Nat-M; Staph.
Bleeding (minor): Arn; Cal; Hyp; Led; Phos.
Bruising: Arn; Ham; Hyp;Led; Ruta.
Burns, minor: Cal; Canth; Phos.
Cuts and grazes: Cal; Hyp; Led; Staph.
Eye trauma (minor): Arg-N; Euphr; Ham; Led; Puls; Ruta.
Headaches/minor head injuries: Arn; Arg-N; Bell; Bry; Eup-P;
Gels; Hyp; Ign; Nat-M; Nux-V; Ruta; Sil.
Fractures (until professionally treated): Arn; Bry; Eup-P; Ruta; Sil.
Muscular-skeletal sprains or strains: Arn; Bry; Led; Puls; Rhus-T;
Ruta.
Puncture wounds: Apis; Arn; Hyp; Led.
Shock, emotional: Arn; Ign.
Shock, physical: Arn, Carb-V.
Sunstroke: Bell; Nat-M.

Acute treatment

The following is a brief definition of levels of severity of acute
cases, and the action which would be appropriate for each. Chronic
conditions and constitutional cases are not appropriate for home
treatment.

The acute case requiring immediate attention

A potentially life-threatening condition, examples of which are: a
traffic accident, a victim of fire or asphyxiation or shock, a possible
case of heart attack or stroke, an asthma attack or other breathing
difficulties, headache accompanied with visual disturbances or a
stiff neck, high fever, inability to urinate, inexplicable bleeding or
great listlessness.

Action: Call the emergency services, ambulance or for other
medical assistance immediately. If, and only if, it will not
exacerbate injuries, give the appropriate homeopathic first aid to
lessen distress, providing it is acceptable to the individual. There
would be no time for elaborate case taking. Practise general first-
aid principles where necessary, if you have this training, and advise
the professionals of your actions when they arrive.

Dose: You may give a single dose of your chosen remedy at 30C if symptoms are intense; or a dose every three minutes with a lower potency (6C or 12C), repeating if the symptoms relapse. You will see improvement if the remedy is well chosen, but it may wear off quickly and need to be repeated, especially at low potencies. It may also need to be altered to another remedy altogether, according to your observations. Give the remedy less frequently once there is a lessening in the severity of the symptoms or an increase in well being and stop altogether when improvement is marked (definite). Stop also if symptoms worsen. This may be evidence of the Laws of Cure. The return of old symptoms are a sign of healing best left alone, they will pass naturally. Worsening symptoms could also indicate that the remedy has triggered the cure unnoticed, and repeats are now initiating aggravation by proving the remedy.

The acute case requiring urgent attention

Non-emergency acute cases start suddenly with great intensity of symptoms at the outset, and probably include severe pain, but although immediate treatment is needed, they are not usually life threatening. The patient will have experienced a rapid loss of equilibrium, and the sense of feeling ill accompanied with symptoms, individually or severally. Examples are severe emotional shock, pain, or an intense fever causing great distress.

Action: In these cases arrange for the person to be seen by a non-emergency healthcare professional as appropriate, and meanwhile give homeopathic first aid to lessen their acute distress.

Dose: Give a single dose at 30C, or alternatively a lower potency such as 6C or 12C two or three times, at intervals of 15 or 30 minutes until improvement occurs, or symptoms reappear. Once a healing reaction is noted increase the time between repeats, allowing up to two hours for the improvement to become marked (or for a relapse), depending on the distress of the patient. Repeat only if necessary (if symptoms are unabated or return, unchanged) up to four times. In any case, pause as soon as a healing response has been triggered and distress is lessened, or if different symptoms present, and stop when positive, marked improvement is felt.

The acute case requiring attention the same day

In these cases the onset is still rapid but the symptoms are less intense than in the previous examples. There may or may not be pain or distress for example, in a case of sickness and diarrhoea following food poisoning.

Action: Depending on the distress of the person you may decide to treat with symptomatic homeopathic first aid, or briefly take the case for a more accurate selection of the remedy.

Dose: Give the chosen remedy at the lower potencies of 6C or 12C for up to six doses at intervals of two hours, repeating only on relapse or when no improvement has been noted. Results should be evident within 24 hours. If well being or an alteration of symptoms is not apparent in that time, try a different remedy; you have probably not selected the correct one at your first attempt. Stop in any case as soon as the healing response has been triggered, or if different symptoms present, or when positive, marked improvement is felt.

The acute minor case

These symptoms could reasonably remain untreated for a few days if necessary, such as a typical heavy cold or muscular pain following over-exertion. Perhaps only TLC (tender, loving care) and time is warranted.

Action: Minor acute symptoms allow you time to take the case properly to identify the single, correct remedy with more care. If you make a remedy selection by traditional homeopathic principles rather than symptomatic first aid, what you learn will stand you in good stead for urgent first-aid situations when they occur. This more professional approach involves questioning the patient if he or she has time, to tease out all the factors which could be relevant for selection of the remedy. We will look at this technique in detail next.

Dose: For mild acute cases try a single dose of 6C or 6X once only, repeating every four to eight hours if there has been no response or if the symptoms relapse. It may take a few days for marked improvement to occur. Improvement may take the form of a desire to sleep, a natural step towards healing in minor conditions, though a potentially alarming one in severe situations.

Traditional homeopathy: taking the case

First impressions

The moment of first meeting your patient or, if the person is already known to you, the moment of the first presentation of a complaint, is of inestimable value. We all learn to present a social face to the world; when to be polite, when it is all right to be vulnerable, when to restrain humour because of the solemnity of a situation, and so on. Such behavioural masks do not necessarily match our inner feelings. It is therefore important to be focused and acutely aware of the person initially seeking your help, to catch the fleeting inner reality which may be glimpsed before the mask of social interaction descends. Health is as much about feeling well as of having no troublesome symptoms. We are also socially encouraged not to be complainers. It is not unusual for a practitioner, when asking how a patient is feeling, to be told, 'Fine, thank you' or 'Not too bad' when pain and discomfort is evident in the patient's attempt to speak, stand or move. This polite reply is uttered from habit, but an observation of the face and body tells a greater truth. Like the person who cleans

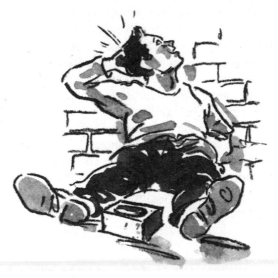

Figure 6   'I am fine ...'

their house because the cleaner is coming today, most of us like to present a favourable self-image and to please those we meet.

So, note body language as well as speech. Note tone as well as words, and above all listen. Listen for the omissions as well as what is said. What is avoided? What might you expect to be mentioned which is not being said? Is the facial rash too embarrassing to state? Is a recent bereavement too painful to discuss? Be tuned to the silences as well as the speech. Is too much said? Does this person have a tendency to exaggeration, or to agree with whatever is suggested? How does the patient look, sound, smell? Are genital or urinary dysfunctions difficult topics for this person to speak of to a relative stranger, a woman, man, a person of a different race or faith? It may be that a gentle enquiry is all the permission this person needs to broach difficult topics. Ask open questions rather than closed ones. An open question such as, 'Can you describe how you feel?' allows for an expansive reply, where a closed one, such as, 'Do you feel hot?' only invites a monosyllabic 'Yes' or 'No'.

Be sure not to lead the answers by asking either/or questions, or suggesting by tone or phrase that you would regard one answer more favourably than another. 'How do you feel?' rather than 'You wouldn't say you were cold, would you?' Mental and emotional symptoms are of the greatest importance as they reveal the subjective experience of the whole patient, but it is not advisable to ask these questions first. To the patient unfamiliar with homeopathic principles, it may seem as if the physical complaint they have come to ask advice for is being dismissed, trivialized or devalued, or that their sanity is in doubt. This could cause withholding, hostility and lack of co-operation. Be wary also of second-guessing the remedy at the point of taking the case. If you suspect Belladonna you might ask questions of the 'Would you say you have a raging fever, are afraid of the curtains and crave lemons' type, to confirm your belief, rather than ask impartial ones which would reveal a different case altogether. A routine format for your questions can prevent lapses of this kind.

The points to cover in your questions

Your questions may surprise the person who has previous experience only of conventional medicine as they enquire into all aspects of the patient's life. You hope to discover any significant changes from what is regarded as normal for this person. If the patient habitually needs only six hours of sleep per night which is a constitutional factor, insomnia is not a symptom of note for the acute case. To treat acute conditions you will need to look for the general symptoms which reflect the state of the whole person, and any unusual or peculiar symptoms. You will pinpoint the correct remedy by the unique symptoms. It is essential that you make notes of your questions and the answers when taking the case history.

Enquire into emotional, physical, mental and general aspects of recent experience. Use your instinct and experience and expand the questions where you sense there is more to be said.

- How are you? Allows for a description in the patient's own words.
- Ask about other family members, and their health patterns. Is there a family history of illness, and if so, what? Is any other family member suffering similar symptoms at present?
- Subjective feelings are usually more distinctive than the location of physical symptoms, so what is the nature of the pain; burning, cramping, pinching, tearing, piercing, stabbing, aching, tingling, for example?
- Is it better or worse at particular time(s) of day or night? Did it start at a particular time?
- How quickly did the symptoms develop?
- Can the onset be linked to any prior situation or activity? Precipitating stress factors are legion and may include weather conditions, diet, emotional news, sleep disruption, anticipated events or pressure of work.
- Was the weather an influence; is it now; is it ever?
- Are the feelings/symptoms eased, or made worse, by action/inaction?
- What else modifies the effect of the symptoms? Are symptoms alleviated or aggravated by alteration of temperature, position, pressure, touch, bathing, sleep, clothing, sound, food, drink, for example? Does altering any of these factors produce a general improvement in well being?

■ Do you crave any particular foods or drinks, or are you repelled by any?

■ Are you perspiring more than usual? Is the sweat localized? Does anything in particular cause you to sweat? Is it a hot or cold sweat?

■ Ask about concentration, memory, tidiness, moods, fears, phobias, reactions to stress, and so on.

■ Did the pain start, or is it located, on one side only or did it move from one side to the other? If so, from which to which?

■ Enquire about changes in sleep patterns, when, how often, in what position, how the patient prefers to be covered, and so on.

■ Remember to enquire whether allopathic medicines are being taken for a chronic condition, as these may have the effect of suppressing symptoms, and may even create new ones. (Orthodox medicines may have caused dis-ease to enter deeper into the body. This would require subtle management by a trained homeopath to reverse the suppressions before the root problem could be addressed.)

■ Remind the patient not to stop orthodox treatments without first asking for advice from the health professional who prescribed them. To do so could be dangerous.

■ Note the absence of symptoms too. If there is a fever without thirst, that is itself extremely noteworthy, as would be chilliness with a refusal to be covered up. These are the sorts of peculiar facts which pinpoint the remedy by their very oddness.

■ See if there are unifying themes to the symptoms, such as an overall tendency towards dryness (of throat, eyes, skin, bowel movements, and so on) or to copious discharges, and, if so, are they of a notable colour or consistency? The colour and nature of discharges can also be very individualizing. You need an overview of the whole person.

In Appendix 3 you will find sample case notes to suggest how you might record the symptoms as you are told them. Many of the common symptoms will be of no use to you, but do not prejudge and fail to record them. You may need to refer back to your notes and may then regret not having taken the case thoroughly. Record keeping is necessary to check on the results of treatment. Keep a note of emotional feelings as well as the physical ones, any conclusions you reach, and note the remedy and the potency (strength) which you recommend, together with the current date. You now have an accurate record should you need to repeat, or alter, the initial remedy, and will know for how long the remedy has been taken. You may well be presented with the return of an acute situation which you know you treated successfully before, but have completely forgotten the remedy and the potency you prescribed, if you fail to keep records. Obviously such records should be kept confidentially. In keeping accurate records you will not only be accumulating a fund of prescribing experience and a useful personal reference source, but your experience may even add to the sum of homeopathic knowledge. You will next need to analyse the notes you have made.

6 | CHARACTERIZING AND THE REPERTORY INDEX

'... they are so much alike – how to distinguish? But get their characteristics and peculiarities of action, and each one stands out distinctly as an entity – almost a personality: and when you have once grasped that personality, and as it were made friends with the drug, you will recognise, as with your friends, not only what he looks like, but his little tricks of manner and speech, how he will behave on all occasions–in regard to noises–foods–friendly overtures–rudeness–sympathy –his restlessness or placidity–his extreme neatness and order, or the opposite–his easy emotion–chilliness–meteoric reactions–his attitude, in short, to environment physical and mental. You will see him in friends and patients, when prescribing becomes comparatively easy, and successful.'

Dr M L Tyler, MD, *Homeopathic Drug Pictures*

Characterizing the case

Now that you have this wealth of information, you need to analyse it to ascertain which single remedy it characterizes from the many in the Materia Medica. Bear in mind that the Materia Medica and Repertory in this volume are necessarily limited, selected with a bias for being commonly found to match symptoms in acute and first-aid situations. The single remedy you seek may be beyond the scope of this work, so if the case you have taken shows strongly individual characteristics not found here, or not coincident with the remainder of the remedy picture where you do find it here, be prepared to research in a larger Materia Medica, or consult a professional. You cannot tailor the symptoms to fit a remedy. The match will be there or it will not.

It is by categorizing the many responses to your questions that you can see the unifying or individualizing pattern which makes selection of the remedy obvious despite the mass of information. What is needed is an overview of the totality of symptoms and a recognition of what is peculiar, special and identifying about this case. Remedies often have a unifying theme which can be detected in the case notes, but beware of reinventing the case with suppositions. How does the patient feel? Subjective experience is the first characteristic to note, so to say, 'I have been feeling tired, but I'm not doing more than usual' would be of particular interest to the homeopath. Make a list which selects only the elements of the case which may help to identify the remedy. To note all the facts which typify a pathology, measles, or fever, for example, would not advance your analysis. Remember it is always the individual person's symptoms which are matched to a remedy. The same remedy is not necessarily given to all cases of a broadly similar disease, though in acute first-aid prescribing it may sometimes seem so. Remember that an infection passed around a family may well lead to several different remedies.

Sort the case notes

Not all symptoms are helpful in selecting the remedy, so your first tasks are to sort and grade them. A common symptom such as an ill-defined headache, even if it is the reason why treatment has been sought, is not useful because it could apply to many remedies equally well. It is the general, individual and peculiar symptoms which are defining. A general symptom is one which affects a person completely, rather than one which is common to many people. An example of a general symptom would be anxiety and depression in someone normally of an even disposition. Nor do you search in the Materia Medica for every symptom in your case notes. This would be a form of pathological prescribing, a treatment of the symptom instead of the person. As cure progresses from the centre outwards and above to below, so symptoms affecting inner, critical organs and the whole being are next in importance, followed by the peculiar symptoms, and last and least, the common and local symptoms. So, you can categorize each of the symptoms according to type

General symptoms

Despite the implied irrelevance of the name, general symptoms are of paramount importance. They apply to the whole individual, and so are general in that sense. They are often subjective, mental or emotional symptoms which are described by the patient prefaced with 'I ...', such as, 'I feel depressed,' but may be physical, such as 'I am burning up all over.' Subjective feelings like this are important because a sense of well being or disease precedes physical changes, whether towards disease or cure. General symptoms affect the whole person deeply.

Peculiar symptoms

Peculiar and unusual symptoms may serve to identify the case if they are characteristic and were recorded by provers of the remedy. These are symptoms which are rarely encountered, or rarely absent, with this sort of case. So, for instance, a fever without thirst is more peculiar than a fever with thirst; and measles without spots is more peculiar than with them. These would be important facts to aid your deliberations. Here you should beware of another pitfall. The apparently odd symptom, on further enquiry, may just be the patient's way of compensating for an irrelevant fact which has not been mentioned. To prefer to sleep on one side may be significant, though if asked why, you might learn it is merely because there is a draught from the door in the bedroom; an irrelevance.

Particular symptoms

In contrast, these apply to specific organs or body parts, such as a cramping stomach pain, or a red face. They are of less use for identifying the remedy but may help to refine a choice if in doubt. Some symptoms can be described as common and particular at the same time. They are those which typically affect particular areas, such as having a sore nose with a cold. Particular symptoms may be the reason why treatment was sought, but they are not necessarily useful for a diagnosis.

Common symptoms

These are usually associated with a particular pathology, or those which would apply to lots of remedies if looked up in the Repertory. They are of little or no use for assessing the acute case and need not be added to your Repertory list or grid. Spots with measles is a common symptom, as is the modality of being better for fresh air.

So, you can collect individual facts by the truckload, but unless you have noted the individualizing characteristics well, you will not be able to select the correct remedy. In the absence of obviously peculiar or individual symptoms you need an overview of the totality of symptoms, which can identify the remedy. This might be a general tendency to dryness or redness; that all discharges are yellow; a general avoidance of change; or extreme rage. There are various ways to eliminate the irrelevant and make such an overview clearer. Two such are the analysis of symptoms by making a list; and the use of a Repertory grid, a method favoured by many homeopaths. I shall briefly explain each of these two methods.

Refine the search (1) – The repertory list

First use the symptoms from your case notes to create a separate Repertory list. The next step will be made easier if you do this in the style that the repertory adopts. Take a look at the Repertory index now (p. 83) if you have not done so before. You will see that symptoms are listed by their nature and location, plus what preceded their appearance and what alters their behaviour. Make your list from your case notes in a similar fashion, so, 'It hurts all over, as if I'm on fire and I am so thirsty. I have been drinking cold water all day' becomes:

Pain, intense, burning
Thirst, great, for cold water

on your list. Leave enough space to enter abbreviations of the relevant remedies beside your notes. The following example shows how your case-taking notes become your repertory list ready for analysis. The patient anxiously says:

'I don't know what is the matter with me. We had a lovely day out yesterday, it was windy but the sun was lovely. It was a treat to be out in the fresh air but today I am in agony.'

■ Precipitated by:
  – exposure to dry winds. Acon, Hep-S.
  – exposure to sun. Acon, Canth, Nat-M.

■ Better for fresh air. Acon, All-C, Arg-N, Arn, Carb-V, Dros, Ip, Lyc, Nat-M, Puls, Sep, Sul.

■ Anxious. Acon, Arn, Ars, Bry, Dros, Eup-P, Lyc, Puls, Sep.

'It hurts all over, as if I'm fire and I am so thirsty. I have been drinking cold water all day.'

■ Pain,
  - intense. Acon.
  - burning. Acon, Apis-Mel, Arn, Ars, Canth, Phos, Sul.

■ Thirst, great, for cold water. Acon, Phos.

'I couldn't stop sneezing this morning.'

■ Sneezing fit, morning. Acon.

'Can you turn that light away, please? It makes my eyes hurt.'

■ Worse for light. Acon, All-C, Bell, Euphr, Phos, Sil.

'I was fine last night.'

■ Onset sudden. Acon, Apis-Mel, Bell, Canth, Hep-S, Ip.

You have a match with *Acon* for all of these symptoms, and only with *Acon* for the sneezing fit. That odd sympton confirms the other generally correct ones. Aconite is suggested here. Your case may not be this simple, but the principles of analysis remain the same.

Grade the symptoms

Some homeopaths also define symptons by their degrees of importance. They may underline general, subjective symptoms three times, particular symptoms twice, and common symptoms once to help when analysing them. Or you might put a triangle around or beside the general keywords, put a square around particular keywords and circle around common keywords, to distinguish them. Whatever way you use to stress the importance of symptoms, enter the general and particular symptoms onto your new list, ignoring the common symptoms. Find the remedies with which they are known to be associated by referring to the Repertory index. Enter all the abbreviated remedies you find for each of your main case symptoms against each symptom on your Repertory list. When you have done this it should be evident which remedies appear repeatedly, and how many times. Add the number of times each remedy appears on your list and enter the scores. There should only be a few remedy abbreviations which coincide often. (If all of them do, you have probably entered common rather than defining symptoms. If none appears more than once you either have a case beyond the scope of this book, or need to reconsider the original note taking.) If you have taken the case well, this will leave just one remedy which matches all of the important symptoms, though others will also match some of them.

Find which is the correct single remedy from among those with high scores in your list by reading the whole entry for each in the Materia Medica. Determine how well the rest of the symptoms match your case. You are unlikely to find any case which matches every possible symptom, but most of the main symptoms should be present in your case. The selection of the remedy should be precise and scientific, so if you miss the important points you will fail to find the remedy which matches.

Large Repertory indexes show the symptom types graded even further, according to the degree of certainty with which this symptom is found with a specific remedy, as established by provings. The grade one symptoms are usually shown in a Repertory in bold type. These were found to occur in every single case of the many people who proved the remedy. The second grade of symptoms, often shown in italics, were found by a high proportion of the provers; and the third grade in normal type were noted sometimes or rarely, or have yet to be confirmed by re-proving.

Refine the search (2) – The Repertory grid

A Repertory grid can be of great help in deciphering your notes to make a meaningful remedy selection from them. I have included an example of a Repertory grid which can be copied for your use (Figure 7). Whatever method you decide to adopt, prepare blank copies so you use the same format on each occasion to keep your method consistent. You can then learn from experience as retrospective assessments and comparisons are made easier and more meaningful. Make consistent case-taking a habit.

REMEDIES

SYMPTOMS	ACONITE	ALLIUM CEPA	APIS MELLIFICA	ARGENT NIT.	ARNICA	ARSENICUM	BELLADONNA	BRYONIA	CALCAREA CARBONICA	CALENDULA	CANTHARIS	CARBO VEG.	CHAMOMILLA	CUPRUM MET.	DROSERA	EUPATORIUM PERFOLIATA	EUPHRASIA	GELSEMIUM	HAMAMELIS	HEPAR SULPH.	HYPERICUM	IGNATIA	IPECAC.	KALI. BICH.	LEDUM PALUSTRE	LYCOPODIUM	MERC.	NAT. MUR.	NUX. VOM.	PHOSPHORUS	PULSATILLA	RHUS. TOX.	RUTA GRAV.	SEPIA	SILICA	STAPHYSAGRIA	SULPHUR
1.																																					
2.																																					
3.																																					
4.																																					
5.																																					
6.																																					
7.																																					
8.																																					
9.																																					
10.																																					
11.																																					
12.																																					
13.																																					
14.																																					
15.																																					
16.																																					
17.																																					
18.																																					
19.																																					
20.																																					
SCORE																																					

Figure 7 A blank repertory grid for your use

Enter symptoms on the grid

You will see that each of the remedies in the Materia Medica is listed vertically across the top of the grid, with numbered black spaces horizontally down the left side. Enter the symptoms from your case-taking in the spaces on the left, one to each line. (See the completed sample grid in Figure 8.) Once the symptoms have been entered, look for the remedies with which they are proven to be associated, by referring to the Repertory index. You will see there are abbreviated remedy names alongside each repertory entry. Enter these remedies on your grid by placing a tick or cross where the remedy concerned meets the line of the symptom concerned. A single symptom may require that you tick several different remedy boxes. If almost every remedy could be ticked it is probably a common symptom of little use in defining the curative remedy you seek. If there are about a dozen or less applicable remedies, mark each one along the symptom line. When all the symptoms have been correlated to possible remedies you should be able to detect a pattern. A few remedies will have a lot of ticks while others have few, or only one. (See the example again.) If you have taken the case exceptionally well a single remedy will have a tick beside every symptom, even though other remedies may also match some of them. It would be unusual to take the case so well to start with, so you will probably need to decide which of a few potential remedies, each with a lot of ticks on the grid, is the correct single one. Add the columns and enter the scores along the bottom line. You may be so accurate in your case taking that there is a clear 'winner'. More likely there will be several contenders. The relative likelihood of each being the correct one should now be obvious. Turn to the Materia Medica for the probable remedies (those with the most ticks), and read the whole symptom picture there. Your case will not match exactly, but if it differs in the key points it is not the correct one. Try the others in the same way. Your case should match the peculiar, unusual and characteristic symptoms that identify the correct remedy. If none does, it may be that your note taking or questioning needs further consideration, or that the remedy which applies to the case before you is not within the scope of this Materia Medica. If you suspect this to be so, you may like to check in a larger volume if you can refer to one, or suggest your patient sees a professional.

SYMPTOMS

1. Precipitated by exposure to dry winds.
2. Precipitated by exposure to sun.
3. Better for fresh air.
4. Anxious.
5. Pain, intense.
6. Pain, burning.
7. Thirst, great, for cold water.
8. Sneezing fit.
9. Worse for light.
10. Sudden onset.
11.
12.
13.
14.
15.
16.
17.
18.
19.
20.

REMEDIES

Remedy	1	2	3	4	5	6	7	8	9	10	SCORE
ACONITE	✓	✓	✓	✓	✓	✓	✓	✓	✓	✓	10
ALLIUM CEPA			✓						✓		2
APIS MELLIFICA							✓			✓	2
ARGENT NIT.		✓		✓							2
ARNICA			✓	✓			✓				3
ARSENICUM			✓	✓							2
BELLADONNA									✓	✓	2
BRYONIA				✓			✓				2
CALCAREA CARBONICA											
CALENDULA											
CANTHARIS	✓					✓			✓		3
CARBO VEG.			✓								1
CHAMOMILLA											
CUPRUM MET.											
DROSERA		✓	✓								2
EUPATORIUM PERFOLIATA		✓	✓								2
EUPHRASIA									✓		1
GELSEMIUM											
HAMAMELIS											
HEPAR SULPH.						✓			✓		2
HYPERICUM											
IGNATIA											
IPECAC.		✓							✓		2
KALI. BICH.											
LEDUM PALUSTRE											
LYCOPODIUM		✓	✓								2
MERC.											
NAT. MUR.	✓	✓									2
NUX. VOM.											
PHOSPHORUS						✓	✓		✓		3
PULSATILLA		✓	✓								2
RHUS. TOX.											
RUTA GRAV.											
SEPIA		✓	✓								2
SILICA									✓		1
STAPHYSAGRIA											
SULPHUR		✓				✓					2

Figure 8 Sample repertory grid

Over time some remedies will become as familiar as if they were friends. Humans have an amazing ability to recognize the features of someone once known, even though they may not have seen them for years. Although most people have two eyes, a nose and a mouth, we can also pick out a known face among others in a crowd. These impressive human attributes can be brought to play on learning the symptom pictures which distinguish one remedy from another. If visualized and memorized as if they were a person, the remedies will become your friends. Once a remedy has been encountered in life a few times you will recognize it as easily as the features on your best friend's face.

It should be obvious now why it is the odd and unusual features of a case which make remedy selection easier. Headache is an aspect of many symptom pictures, and alone is not a good identifier of a remedy. However, if it is an unusual headache in some way, starting on one side of the head followed by the other, for instance, it could help you to identify the remedy for the whole symptom picture. Similarly, there are so many possible symptoms which may accompany the common cold, for instance, that although this is the complaint you are asked to treat, it may not be the cold symptoms which will identify the whole remedy picture. Remember there is only ever one state of disease in a person at one time, however varied the symptoms of the resulting imbalance. Remember each person has a unique response to stress, so among the common cold symptoms you hope to identify the rare, the particular or the general symptoms which describe *this* person's case.

Administer the remedy

Armed with the single remedy to match your patient's symptom picture you must now decide on the appropriate dose, potency and frequency, and explain to the patient how the remedy should be administered, stored and handled. It is standard practice in classical homeopathy to prescribe and note the reaction to a single remedy and to prescribe another only when you are sure that the first has shown itself to be ill-matched to the symptom picture. This could happen several times with a single case while you are learning. If nothing has happened after a reasonable time, you should reassess your selection from your notes, your list or grid, and the Materia Medica.

There is a real risk of exacerbating the person's condition when dabbling with chronic cases. If the similimum to the acute case has been found, all the symptoms should improve over time, though if any were suppressed they will reappear on their way to cure. When one symptom is treated only to be replaced by another, then that is treated, but yet another appears, and so on, all that is achieved is the re-suppression of symptoms, which is not good homeopathic practice. Treatment of this kind will drive the root problem deeper within the body where it will manifest different, perhaps more critical, symptoms and make the true similimum harder to identify.

Visit a professional homeopath

It is a good idea to learn the thoroughness of a professional approach even if you only expect to treat minor conditions. When prescribing for yourself, for instance, it is almost impossible to be entirely objective even with the best of intentions. You may believe that you did not sleep all night, but if asked, your partner would describe being kept awake by your snores. Likewise, you might be quite unaware of changes in your mood which are apparent to others and of course, if you, or anyone else, have a chronic condition requiring a constitutional remedy you really should seek professional advice.

If you are serious about learning to treat others homeopathically, it is sensible to have experienced the method first hand, if only to check your self-diagnosis. The experience will be a valuable part of your learning process. Select someone who can give evidence of reputable training and qualifications. Ask what the charges will be. Different practitioners do charge different rates, sometimes due to the very high demand for their services, or perhaps for the higher costs of their well-located premises. Decide whether you feel comfortable with the practitioner you select. Remember you will be discussing many intimate aspects of your life with this person, and may be advised to make lifestyle changes by them. If you do not feel a rapport, or might resist advice, try another practitioner.

The fee is usually higher for the first visit than for subsequent ones. This is reasonable since taking note of your case details may take approximately two hours. Once you have been prescribed a remedy your following visit(s) will be shorter, and should be less expensive. Remember that, in most cases, if the remedy is well chosen it will trigger a reaction quickly. Chronic or constitutional treatments can continue for weeks, months or years in some cases, however some remedies take effect immediately. Many practitioners allow a brief consultation without charge so that you can learn about their methodology (ask if it will be constitutional or pathological/symptomatic treatment), discuss fees, establish rapport, and give some idea of your problem before an appointment is made. Many practitioners also have explanatory brochures or leaflets to take home, so you can decide whether to proceed with an appointment or not without any pressure.

7 | HOW TO TAKE THE MEDICINE

Whatever the method of application, the remedy should not be touched directly, as this can nullify its effect. This can be achieved by tipping the dose into the lid or a spoon to transport it to the mouth. Pillules or tablets should be placed under the tongue or against the inner cheek to dissolve. Saliva provides fast absorbtion of the remedy by the body and allows the body to respond naturally. If the patient finds taking these small hard pills difficult, the pharmacist can prepare soft tablets, globules which are as small as poppy seeds, or powders by request.

Internal remedies

Powders may be taken as they are, or dissolved in water. Pills or pillules may be crushed between two spoons or dissolved in a small glass of water, in which case the patient should take a teaspoonful of the remedy at the prescribed frequency. (Each spoonful amounts to a complete application of the remedy, not a fraction of it.) If the patient cannot tolerate cows' milk (which sac lac tablets are made of), it is possible to take the remedy prepared in liquid form, in which case a few drops may be taken neat, or added to a glass of water, or in the form of sucrose, which as plain sugar is easily transported and taken. The carrier used for liquid remedies then is alcohol or water rather than saccharum lactose, the cows' milk derivative. A few pharmacies are able to prepare the remedies in rice wafer form for those unable to tolerate milk or sugar. Fortunately such preparations are easily mailed and so may still be obtained even if the local pharmacists cannot oblige.

If you decide to recommend or use tinctures, they should never be taken orally.

External remedies

Remedies for external use have yet to be subjected to the rigorous proving of the internal remedies. Creams and ointments are prepared as far as possible to homeopathic principles. Calendula is one such and is invaluable for the promotion of rapid healing without scars and the prevention of sepsis.

Concerning the frequency of remedy application

There are really no homeopathic doses, only complete remedies, so it is incorrect to think of repeating a remedy until a sufficient dose produces the healing effect. Each time a remedy is repeated, the whole remedy is given, not a part of it, although it is referred to as a dose. Thus each drop in a vial and each pillule in the container is the whole remedy. If the condition is acute, the remedy well chosen, and the patient sensitive to its action, the single dose could be all that is required. Some patients whose susceptibility is reduced or who are suffering extremely acute symptoms, as when injured, in high fever, great pain or aroused emotions, or who might have benefitted by a higher potency, may benefit by repeating the remedy, having allowed a reasonable time for the action of the first dose. You should not repeat remedies routinely, and must never do so when the patient is improving, or when Hering's Laws of Cure is in progress (the reappearance of symptoms in the reverse of the order in which they first occurred). Give a remedy until improvement occurs, then at greater intervals than before until a marked reaction is noted, and then stop.

How soon to repeat the remedy will depend on the potency and severity of symptoms, but always hesitate rather than repeat a remedy carelessly. In non-acute cases you might wait days, or weeks, while in an acute emergency situation, only a few minutes. To continue doses after definite improvement may cause the aggravation or suppression of symptoms, but will not remove symptoms if the remedy is ill-matched. Observe reactions closely, and stop as soon as a definite reaction is noted, or if you doubt your choice. Never alter the remedy to another if a discharge is triggered; consult a professional. If there is no reaction to a given remedy after two or three applications, reconsider, select a closer match to the symptoms and give a different remedy, having discontinued the former one. At the low potencies suggested no harm will have been done. This re-evaluation may become necessary several times until you become more adept at recognizing the key symptoms which identify the correct remedy. The frequency of administration is determined by how acute the symptoms are. The more acute the condition, the more frequently the remedy is repeated until vitality improves and symptoms subside or change. In an acute emergency case it may be necessary to repeat the remedy every five minutes for three applications at low potency, or a single dose of a higher potency. Usually acute conditions respond to the correct remedy within seconds, though they may relapse and require a repeat dose. Stop as soon as the healing response is triggered (when the patient says he or she feels better, as well as by any observable remission of symptoms). The presenting symptoms in severe, non-acute conditions will be a case of less urgent pain than acute ones, with a less sudden onset. They may require two or three applications every 15 or 30 minutes, repeating as necessary every one to two hours, until an effect is noted or another remedy seems indicated. Remember that you should give only one remedy at a time.

Generally, the more acute the symptoms or situation, the more rapid will be the response. The remedy should be allowed time to take effect before a repeat remedy is given, or a different one is tried and dosage should be stopped once a definite improvement is noted. A sense of greater well being may be expressed before the symptoms abate. This is enough cause to stop the remedy, or at least lengthen the period between repeats. Remember, in homeopathic treatment the aim is to trigger the body's response to healing, and healing progresses according to the Laws of Cure. It is the body, rather than heavy medication, which restores health. Sleep is often the first sign of improvement. If the condition improves and well being is experienced, only for a relapse to occur at a later time, you may restart the remedy but be sure the symptoms are exactly as before. It could be that a different remedy is indicated now. Experience and common sense will enable you to determine the distinction between degrees of severity. If you are carefully noting the symptoms and the patient's description of their onset, and improvement, the difference should be apparent.

Two cautionary factors when prescribing

1 Allopathic medicine is the more prevalent method of treatment in most parts of the world. Amateur homeopaths should be alert to the possibility of an acquired, unintentional tendency to treat symptoms, rather than treat the whole person, when prescribing homeopathic remedies. If the symptoms are ill-matched to a remedy it is possible to drive the problem to deeper levels, and create problems which will require professional help to reverse. The principles of homeopathy require that the person is treated and not their symptoms. Fortunately suppression of this kind does not happen very often. The greatest risk of causing suppression is in treating chronic, systemic dis-ease symptoms such as accompany acne, eczema, asthma and diabetes mellitus. Eczema symptoms may be successfully lifted only to create the problem of asthma at a deeper level. These more constitutional conditions should be professionally treated to avoid making the situation worse.

2 If a patient continues to take a homeopathic remedy after a curative response has been triggered, it is possible to actually prove the remedy instead. (Proving results in the production of the symptoms associated with the remedy, leading to greater imbalance and dis-ease than was experienced before starting to take the remedy, even if there was initially some improvement.) If this should happen, it may be counteracted by deliberate antidoting. To do this one should take the substances normally avoided when taking a homeopathically prepared remedy, such as strong coffee, preferably without milk or cream for maximum effect, though this will not work for everyone.

Alternative antidotes are: Camphor, if used externally, as by exposure to the scent of mothballs, or application of penetrating camphor based muscle ointments; peppermint, taken in the form of sweets or a herbal tea. Even minty toothpaste or chewing gum can act as an antidote; menthol or eucalyptus, whether taken internally as cough sweets or a cough mixture, or externally applied as a chest rub, oil or balm. Alcohol also acts as an antidote. Antidotes are generally the substances to avoid while taking a homeopathic remedy, but in the case of accidental provings caused by overdose, they can be useful. However, having turned back the clock to the pre-remedy situation, the original, uncomplicated condition will still remain and need more accurate treatment.

Handling and storage

Remedies are easily contaminated by contact, so try not to touch them directly. If a remedy is taken soon after eating spicy food, drinking black tea, coffee or alcohol, or smoking it may be antidoted and become ineffectual. This is particularly noticeable if a remedy has been working but ceases after exposure to any of these items. Generally, unless taken to excess, the remedy would still work, but if it fails it is worth considering whether it has been antidoted. If so, wait for 30 minutes if the condition is not too acute, then try the remedy again. Exposure of the remedies to strong-smelling agents will also antidote them, in this case, irreversibly. Such remedies should be discarded and replaced. As the healing response initiated by a remedy can remain effective in the body for days, weeks or months, it is recommended that you avoid exposure to strong tasting or smelling substances for at least a month after taking homeopathic treatment. There are many acceptable alternatives to caffeine based drinks and minty toothpastes or mouthwashes available which will not interfere with your remedy. Take advice from your local wholefood supplier.

8 | EVALUATE THE RESULTS

Recognize reaction to the remedy

The patient who has a healing response will usually begin to feel better, perhaps even before the symptoms begin to subside. There are occasions, however, when the initial reaction indicates the body needs to rid itself of suppressed emotion, stress or toxins causing increased tiredness, weepiness, or diarrhoea. This could be the first sign of a successful reaction to the remedy if such symptoms are shortlived. Diarrhoea should not be allowed to continue for more than 24 hours without intervention, less for an infant, because of the risk of dehydration. Generally the patient should be encouraged to honour the demands of the body and rest if tired, or find a comfortable means to acknowledge grief, if it is felt. However, if these cleansing reactions are protracted, you should seek professional advice. It could be that they are new symptoms unconnected with the remedy which indicate a worsening of the condition. In this situation the patient should be referred to a doctor or qualified homeopath for advice.

You should therefore closely observe the patient for changes in mood and levels of vitality as well as for the alleviation or aggravation of symptoms which will dictate when it is time to stop prescribing. Look for a relaxation of former anxieties or fever, a calmer response to questions, or a lapse into peaceful sleep as indicators of a successful healing response.

Some patterns of illness, such as measles, have a commonly observed tendency to trigger different symptoms as stages of healing progress, each stage suggestive of a different remedy. If treating a condition known to exhibit common stages, you may give successive remedies according to the patient's progressive symptom picture. However, do stop repeating and revising remedies once a greater sense of well being is expressed by the patient and improvement is noted.

Aggravations

Remember that a sign of healing may be the temporary worsening of symptoms in some instances. In short-term acute conditions aggravation may merely be evidence that the remedy has effectively stimulated the body. The reaction will be short lived and is not necessarily reason for concern. If the reaction is extreme, it may indicate a chronic condition where tissue changes have occurred, indicating an aggravation of the disease, rather than a harmless brief aggravation of the symptoms. If improvement does not follow aggravated symptoms after allowing a sensible period for them to subside, refer to a professional for advice. Do not continue to prescribe the same remedy, nor try to counterbalance its effects. This will only further complicate the symptom picture, and make the professional's work of triggering of a healing response more difficult.

The sort of aggravation likely to be encountered are a rise in the patient's temperature, when reduction of it is sought; aggravated itching; increased agitation; or vomiting due to heightened nausea, and a weakening of the person while the symptoms strengthen. Do not routinely assume that you are witnessing a temporary aggravation. As a responsible homeopath you should be constantly re-evaluating the situation. If in doubt, get help. Bear in mind that a worsening of symptoms may be a sign that the dis-ease process is progressing unchecked because the wrong remedy was given. Learn to recognize when professional help should be sought. If you place your need for respect above your patient's welfare, both will suffer. You will gain increased respect, trust and gratitude by exercising wise humility when the situation demands it.

9 THE HOME FIRST AID CHEST

If stored carefully, homeopathic remedies can remain effective for many years. For correct storage, keep them in a cool, dark place where they will not get damp. They should be in airtight containers well away from anything which could taint by its smell. Strong-smelling substances contaminate and antidote homeopathic remedies, so avoid placing them near camphor, eucalyptus, muscular heat treatments or other such medicines, chest rubs, cough mixtures, perfumes, bath essences and household cleaners. If exposed to such influences the remedies should be discarded and replaced. Because the remedies remain effective if stored well (hundred-year-old remedies have been found to still effect a cure) it is a good idea to create a collection of the remedies most likely to be called upon in the event of sudden illness or accident in and around the home. For the treatment of accidents, injuries and minor ailments consider: Acon, Apis Mel, Arn, Ars, Bell, Bry, Cal, Canth, Cham, Eup-P, Gels, Hep-S, Hyp, Led, Merc, Nat-M, Nux-V, Puls, Rhus-T, Ruta, Sil, Staph, Sul.

Be aware of the conditions which are beyond the scope of amateur treatment. You should always get medical assistance for urgent situations, though homeopathic remedies may safely relieve immediate shock while help is on the way. This includes all chronic diseases, treatment early in pregnancy and to very young babies. Though all can respond well to homeopathy, I suggest that in these cases prescribing should be left to professionals. The treatment of chronic conditions, babies, newly pregnant women and nursing mothers should be left to professionals, as should emergency situations which might need additional orthodox medical intervention. A course of general first-aid procedures, such as resuscitation methods, recovery positions, and dealing with crisis situations effectively, will benefit your family and assist you to cope with whatever acute problems you may encounter. I also recommend a basic course in homeopathic treatment such as is found in many local education establishments.

10 THE REPERTORY: KEY TO THE MATERIA MEDICA

abscesses *Calc-C, Hep-S, Merc, Sil*
affectionate *Phos, Puls.*
agitated *Acon*
allergic reactions *Apis Mel*
anaemia *Calc-C, Nat-M, Phos, Puls, Staph, Sul.*
anger *Apis Mel, Arn, Ars, Bell, Bry, Canth, Cham, Dros, Hep-S, Ign, Ip, Lyc, Nat-M, Nux-V, Phos, Sep, Staph*
anguish *Ign*
anxious *Acon, Arg-N, Arn, Ars, Bell, Bry, Dros, Eup-P, Lyc, Puls, Sep*
  anticipatory and pre-performance anxiety *Arg-N, Lyc*
  control, must have, *Ars*
  needless, *Lyc*
  untidyness causes, *Ars*
  woken in the night, causes, *Ars*
apathetic *Nat-M, Phos, Puls, Sep, Staph*
apperance, general
  aged prematurely *Lyc*
  droops *Sep, Sul*
  forehead, deep lines in *Lyc*
  redness *Acon, Bell, Sul*
    of face *Apis Mel, Bell, Cham, Euphr*
    spots *Sul*
    streaks *Bell*
  shoulders, raised *Eup-P*
  slouches when erect *Sul*
  slumped when sitting *Sul*
  unkempt, uncaring about *Sul*
appetite, concerning *Arg-N, Calc-C, Cupr, Ign, Lyc, Nux-V, Sul*
  disrupted *Arg-N, Ign, Nux-V*
  eating disorders *Ign*
  hunger followed by aversion to food *Cupr*
  midmorning *Sul*
  large *Calc-C*
  loss of *Lyc*
aversion to
  airless room *Sul*
  attention *Cham*
  food, sight or smell of *Ars*
  foods
    bread *Nat-M, Puls*
    cheeses, strong *Sul*
    dairy foods *Staph*
    coffee *Calc-C*
    eggs *Sul*
    fatty foods *Carb-V, Hep-S, Puls*
    fruit *Ign*
    hot food or drinks *Phos, Puls*
    meat *Calc-C, Sep, Sil, Sul*
    milk *Calc-C, Carb-V, Ign, Staph*
    rich and spicy foods *Merc*
    salt *Merc*
    sweets and candies *Merc*

fresh air   *Ign*
light   *Canth, Euphr*
solitude   *Lyc*
touch   *Acon, Apis Mel, Cham*
washing   *Sul*
wet, becoming accidentally   *Puls*
weather, wet and windy   *Puls*

back ache *see* **Pains**
bedcovers
cannot bear weight of an
affected part   *Ruta*
cause uneasiness   *Sep*
rejected, yet wakes feeling cold
Puls
bedwetting, if unusual   *Puls*
belching   *Arg-N, Carb-V, Lyc,
Nat-M*
loud   *Arg-N*
bereavement, sense of loss   *Acon,
Gels, Ign, Nat-M, Puls, Staph*
better for… *see* **Modalities**
bites and stings (animal or insect)
*Arn, Apis Mel, Canth, Hyp,
Led*
immediately following   *Arn*
infected, swollen, painful to the
touch   *Led*
inflamed   *Hyp*
itchy, shiny and red swelling
Apis Mel
mosquito   *Led*
nerves affected   *Hyp*
bleeding, nature of   *Ham, Phos*
bleeding internally (bruised)
Ham
bright red blood   *Phos*
dark blood after injury, dental
treatment, childbirth   *Ham*
easily, profusely, slow to
coagulate   *Phos*
blisters
itchy   *Rhus-T*

on tongue   *Nat-M*
bloated with gas   *Lyc, Nux-V, Sul*
bones   *Arn, Eup-P, Ruta, Sil*
ache as if broken   *Eup-P*
broken   *Arn, Ruta*
slow to heal   *Sil*
painful   *Ruta*
bored, becomes easily   *Hep-S*
breath, offensive   *Calc-C, Carb-
V, Hep-S, Merc, Puls, Sul*
sour smelling   *Hep-S*
breathing *see* **respiration**
broody   *Nat-M*
bruises   *Arn, Ham, Hyp, Led, Ruta*
around the eye (black eye) which
affects sight   *Ham, Led*
burns and scalds, minor   *Arn,
Cal, Canth*
before emergence of blisters
Canth
burning pain *see* **Pain**

caesarian section, following   *Cal,
Hyp, Staph*
capricious   *Merc*
catarrh   *Eup-P, Euphr, Hep-S,
Kali-B, Merc, Sil, Sul*
alternates with diarrhoea or
rheumatic joint pains   *Kali-B*
catheterization, after   *Staph*
change, symptoms
constantly   *Cupr, Puls, Ign, Ip,
Merc*
cyclic   *Ip*
variable but in a pattern   *Cupr,
Ign*
worse for *see* **Modalities**
childbirth   *Acon, Arn, Cal, Cham,
Ham, Hyp, Staph*
during labour, pains of   *Cham*
following   *Acon, Arn, Cal,
Staph*
leading to haemorrhoids   *Ham*

chills, feeling of   *Euphr, Eup-P, Gels, Ip, Led, Merc, Nux-V*
at 7–9 am   *Eup-P*
despite fever   *Gels, Nux-V*
following feeling of bone ache   *Eup-P*
with great fever   *Gels*
violent   *Ip*
chilly type   *Ars, Calc-C, Euphr, Hep-S, Kali-B, Led, Lyc, Puls, Sep, Sil*
cold, icy   *Sil*
but rejects all warmth   *Puls*
resistant to warmth   *Sil*
sensitive to cold yet needs fresh air   *Ars*
circulation, poor   *Calc-C, Carb-V, Sep*
cold hands and feet   *Sep*
with weakness, blue extremities and cold skin   *Carb-V*
claustrophobia   *Arg-N*
clingy, when ill   *Puls*
collapse   *Carb-V*
common cold/influenza   *All-C, Ars, Calc-C, Eup-P, Gels, Hep-S, Ip, Kali-B, Lyc, Nat-M, Nux-V, Phos*
easily susceptible to   *Ars, Calc-C, Hep-S, Kali-B, Nat-M, Nux-V*
influenza   *Gels*
nasal congestion   *Cal-C, Gels, Ip, Sul*
alternates with watery discharge   *Nat-M, Phos*
dry crusty discharge   *Lyc, Sul*
severe   *Rhus-T*
sneezy, runny nose   *Euphr, Nat-M, Nux-V*
alternates with dry, crusty nasal passages   *Phos*

with chesty cough   *Carb-V*
complains   *Apis Mel, Arg-N, Arn, Ars, Bell, Bry, Cham, Cupr, Hep-S, Ign, Ip, Phos, Puls, Ruta, Sul*
concentration impaired   *Dros, Lyc, Kali-B, Nux-V, Sil*
conceptualizes, but does not realize schemes   *Sul*
concussion   *Arn, Hyp*
confidence lacking, but hides lack   *Lyc*
confused   *Bry, Canth, Gels, Merc, Nat-M*
constipation   *Bry, Calc-C, Gels, Ip, Lyc, Nux-V, Sil, Sul*
alternates with diarrhoea   *Arg-N*
control
controlled exterior while inwardly upset   *Nat-M*
loses   *Bell, Ign, Nux-V*
cough   *Acon, All-C, Bell, Carb-V, Cupr, Dros, Eup-P, Euphr, Hep-S, Ign, Ip, Kali-B, Lyc, Nat-M, Nux-V, Phos, Rhus-T*
absent at night   *Euphr*
choking   *Acon*
coughing fit causes spasms, gasping, shortage of breath   *Cupr, Ign*
dry   *Acon, Bell, Dros, Eup-P, Hep-S, Ip, Lyc, Nux-V*
unable to cough up mucus   *Ip*
hacking, worse for fresh air   *Phos*
loose, productive   *Euphr, Hep-S*
with nausea   *Ip*
nosebleed, precipitated by   *Dros*
painful   *Dros, Eup-P*

persistent
  dry coughing fits, leads to
    gasping for air   *Ip*
  makes eyes water   *Nat-M*
spasmodic   *Dros*
tickly   *Hep-S, Lyc, Nat-M,
  Nux-V, Rhus-T*
violent   *Carb-V*
  child turns blue from   *Ip*
vomiting, caused by   *Dros*
wheezy, dry   *Kali-B*
whooping (pertussis)   *Dros*
cramps   *Cupr*
craves/desires
  affection   *Puls*
  comforting, more in evening
    Puls
  company   *Phos*
  drink, to
    acidic drinks   *Hep-S*
    alcoholic drinks   *Carb-V,
      Staph*
    but worse for   *Led*
    cold drinks, great thirst for
      Acon, Arg-N, Phos,
    milk
      cold   *Rhus-T*
      hot   *Hyp*
    stimulants
      coffee   *Carb-V*
      tea   *Carb-V*
    water, cold, sips as cannot
      tolerate more   *Ars*
  eat, to
    acidic food   *Hep-S*
    butter, despite aversion to
      fatty foods   *Puls*
    chalk   *Calc-C*
    coal   *Calc-C*
    eggs   *Calc-C*
    fats   *Arg-N, Sul*
    food, any, great hunger   *Phos*

highly seasoned foods   *Sul*
meat   *Staph*
pickles, sour foods   *Sep*
raw, hard to digest foods   *Ign*
salt   *Arg-N, Carb-V, Nat-M*
  salty food despite great thirst
    Nat-M
spicy foods, though they upset
  digestion   *Nux-V*
sweets, candies   *Arg-N,
  Calc-C, Carb-V, Lyc, Sep,
  Staph, Sul*
please, to   *Phos, Puls*
  but this exhausts   *Phos*
right, to be   *Lyc*
sleep   *Eup-P*
solitude   *Bry, Gels, Ign, Nat-M,
  Sep*
  if tearful   *Nat-M*
warmth   *Eup-P*
critical, of others   *Apis Mel, Ars,
  Bry, Dros, Hep-S, Ip, Kali-B,
  Ruta*
cuts and lacerations   *Acon, Bell,
  Cal, Hyp, Led, Nux-V, Phos,
  Staph*
  where tissues torn aprt   *Staph*
  wounds which heal slowly   *Sil*
cystitis   *Canth, Staph (see also
  larger Materia Medica)*
  after coitus   *Staph*
  when not urinating   *Staph*

delirious   *Bell*
  with anxiety when feverish
    Rhus-T
demanding   *Hep-S, Ip*
denial, in, (of illness)   *Arn*
depressed   *Arn, Ars, Eup-P, Gels,
  Lyc, Merc, Nat-M, Rhus-T,
  Ruta, Sep*
  on waking   *Lyc*
  weary and   *Ruta*

with a winter cold   *Eup-P*
without clear cause   *Rhus-T*
without weeping   *Gels*
desires *see* **Craves**
despondent   *Carb-V, Sep*
despairing   *Calc-C*
detached and unemotional when
     well   *Sep*
development
  baby rejects mother's milk   *Sil*
  disobedient and wilful child
     Calc-C
  exhaustion in youth, after growth
     spurt   *Phos*
  growth, walking, talking delayed
       in children   *Calc-C, Nat-M*
     fontanelle slow to close   *Sil*
     teething, slow   *Sil*
diarrhoea   *Arg-N, Ars, Calc-C,*
     Cham, Gels, Ip, Nat-M, Nux-
     V, Phos, Sil, Staph, Sul
  after emotional intensity   *Gels*
  alternates with constipation
     Arg-N
  blood streaked, though pain free
     Phos
  copious, watery   *Nat-M*
  food poisoning   *Ars*
  milk, after drinking   *Sil*
  offensive   *Ars, Cham, Sul*
  stools, green   *Ip*
  urgent in the early morning   *Sul*
  watery   *Nat-M*
  with colic   *Staph*
digestion   *Arg-N, Bry, Carb-V,*
     Lyc, Nat-M, Nux-V, Puls, Sil
  baby rejects mother's milk   *Sil*
  bowel, distended, gaseous
     Nat-M
  dyspepsia and flatulence   *Carb-V,*
     Lyc, Nux V
  which is relieved by belching

Carb-V
  heartburn or indigestion   *Arg-N,*
     Nux-V
  metabolism sluggish   *Calc-C,*
     Sep
  poor   *Lyc, Nat-M*
  soon replete or loss of appetite
     Lyc
  upset   *Bry, Nux-V, Puls*
     after eating rich or fatty food
       Puls
discharges   *All-C, Arg-N, Ars,*
     Euphr, Hep-S, Ip, Kali-B, Lyc,
     Nat-M, Phos, Puls, Sil, Sul
  bland   *Puls*
  blood-stained discharges   *Ip,*
     Merc, Phos, Rhus-T, Sil
  ears, from   *Sil*
  eyes, from   *Arg-N, Euphr*
     stinging, watery   *Euphr*
     watery   *Euphr*
  excoriating   *Rhus-T*
  green   *Ip, Merc, Puls*
  mucus   *Ip, Kali-B, Lyc, Sep*
     bloody   *Ip*
     jellified or stringy   *Kali-B*
     profuse   *Kali-B*
     salty and yellow   *Lyc*
     white   *Sep*
     yellow   *Lyc, Sep*
  nose, from   *All-C, Euphr, Kali-B*
     bland   *Euphr*
     burning   *All-C*
     dries in cold air to be replaced
       with headache   *Kali-B*
     dry and crusty, returns if
       removed   *Kali-B*
     worse one side   *All-C*
  profuse   *Euphr, Merc*
     and smelly   *Hep-S*
     and yellow   *Kali-B, Merc*
  salty, yellow   *Lyc, Sep*

smells offensive   *Hep-S, Merc,
  Sil, Sul*
  ears, from, *Sil*
  sores and infections which
    Merc
  sour and cheesy   *Hep-S*
  sputum, bloody   *Ip, Phos*
  suppressed   *Sil*
  thick   *Merc, Nat-M, Puls, Sil*
    green-yellow, all   *Puls*
      causes sores   *Merc*
    yellow   *Puls, Sil*
  thin   *Ars, Merc, Nat-M*
    which burns   *Ars, Merc*
  white   *Nat-M*
  yelloe   *Puls*
dislikes *see* **Aversion to**
dissatisfied, easily   *Ars, Hep-S,
  Merc, Ruta*
distrusts others   *Kali-B, Ruta*
  imagines is being excluded   *Puls*
  imagines slights   *Nux-V*
  reluctant to delegate, though
    busy   *Nux-V*
disturbed   *Bell, Cham*
dizziness   *Nux-V, Rhus-T, Sep*
  feels faint   *Sep*
  sometimes affecting balance
    Rhus-T
dreams, anxiety, nightmares   *Ars,
  Cham, Ign, Led, Nat-M, Rhus-T*
  daydreams   Sul
dryness   *Acon, Bry, Nat-M, Staph,
  Sul*
  coughing fits   *Ip*
  eyes, of   *Staph*
  inflammations   *Bell*
  lips, of   *Bry, Nat-M, Sul*
  mouth, of   *Bry, Nat-M*
  mucous membranes, of   *Bry*
  skin, of   *Nat-M, Sul*

earache, very sensitive to cold air
  Cham, Hep-S
  worse on left side   *Kali-B*
ears   *Cham, Hep-S, Ign, Kali-B,
  Lyc, Nux-V, Rhus-T, Sil*
  congested   *Lyc*
  deafness   *Ign*
  deep itch beyond reach, relieved
    by swallowing   *Nux-V*
  inner, infections of, better for
    yawning   *Sil*
  ringing sound in   *Rhus-T*
  roaring sounds in   *Ign*
  sensation of water in   *Ign*
eating/sleeping patterns, disturbed,
  see **Appetite**
eats rapidly   *Hep-S*
  what knows will cause
    digestive upset   *Puls*
emotional outbursts   *Ign, Nat-M,
  Sep, (see also* **Anger**, **Tearful**,
  etc)
  erractic   *Nat-M*
  inappropraite, misplaced   *Nat-M*
  raving   *Bell*
empathetic   *Phos*
  to needs of animals   *Puls*
evasive   *Hep-S*
excess, of anything   *Nux-V, Staph*
  overwork   *Nux-V*
  sexual intercourse, of   *Staph*
excitable   *Bell, Canth*
extremities
  ache   *Dros*
  blue, with weakness and cold
    skin   *Carb-V*
  cold   *Bell, Euphr, Gels*
  feet hot, especially at night   *Sul*
exhaustion   *Arn, Ars, Calc-C,
  Carb-V, Cupr, Eup-P, Gels, Ip,
  Kali-B, Lyc, Merc, Nat-M,
  Phos, Ruta, Sep, Sil*

alternates with jerking spasms
  Cupr
attempts to please others, when
  Phos
energetic exercise improves,
  despite   *Sep*
extreme   *Gels*
following respiratory illness,
  measles, whooping cough
  Carb-V
listless, tired   *Arn, Eup-P, Gels,
  Kali-B, Lyc, Nat-M, Ruta*
mental   *Cupr*
minor effort produces   *Merc,
  Nat-M*
other symptoms alternate in
  regular cycles with   *Ip*
rapid onset of   *Calc-C*
tired by mental endeavour
  Calc-C, Sil
with restlessness   *Ars*
youthful, following growth spurt
  Phos

eye lids
heavy lidded   *Gels*
inflamed, swollen   *Euphr*
styes   *Staph*

eyes   *All-C, Arg-N, Bell, Bry,
  Eup-P, Euphr, Gels, Led, Lyc,
  Nat-M, Ruta, Sep, Staph, Sul*
ache   *Eup-P*
bloodshot after injury   *Led*
burn   *All-C, Sul*
catarrhal   *Lyc*
dark ringed   *Sep*
glassy   *Gels*
gritty   *Sul*
headache affecting   *Nat-M*
pain behind   *Bry*
pupils dilated   *Bell, Gels*
red   *Led, Ruta, Sul*
sore, gritty, burning, red   *Sul*

staring and glassy   *Bell, Gels*
sticky in morning but dislikes
  washing them   *Sul*
strained, weak, red   *Ruta*
sunken, dry   *Staph*
watery   *All-C, Euphr*

face   *Acon, Apis Mel, Arn, Ars,
  Bry, Calc-C, Cham, Cupr,
  Dros, Euphr, Gels, Ip, Lyc,
  Nat-M, Phos, Puls, Sep, Sul*
blotchy-red   *Phos*
blue and reddened, or pale when
  difficulty breathing   *Ip*
bridge of nose yellow   *Sep*
eyes, dark ringed   *Sep*
flushed   *Phos, Puls*
hot   *Arn, Ars, Dros*
  to the touch, rest of body cold
    Ars
  while extremities cold   *Arn,
    Dros*
mouth   *Ars, Nat-M, Puls* (*see
    also* **Lips, Tongue**)
  dry   *Puls*
  saliva, absent   *Nat-M*
    with bitter taste   *Ars*
  sores around after exposure to
    sun   *Nat-M*
pale appearance   *Acon, Arn,
    Calc-C, Cupr, Ip, Lyc*
  after effort   *Acon*
  as if suffering   *Ars*
  deeply lined, and   *Lyc*
purple   *Gels*
red   *Acon, Apis Mel, Arn, Bry,
    Cham, Euphr, Gels, Ip, Nat-M,
    Phos, Sul*
yellow   *Sep*

fears   *Acon, Arg-N, Ars, Apis Mel,
    Calc-C, Carb-V, Gels, Lyc,
    Nux-V, Phos, Ruta, Rhus-T*

air travel, of, for lack of fresh air and movement   *Rhus-T*

being alone, of   *Ars, Lyc*

criticism, of   *Nux-V*

crowded places, of   *Arg-N, Gels*

dark, of the   *Carb-V, Gels, Phos*

death, of   *Acon, Ars, Phos, Ruta*

doubts will get well again   *Ars*

easily frightened or offended child   *Calc-C*

examinations, of   *Gels*

failure, of   *Arg-N, Lyc*

heights, of   *Arg-N*

humiliation, of   *Lyc*

judgement, of   *Lyc*

loss of control, of   *Ars*

medical assistance when ill, of   *Arn*

morbid   *Ruta*

observation when urinating, of, at any age   *Nat-M*

occult phenomena, of   *Carb-V*

others' motives, of   *Rhus–T*

public speaking, of   *Gels, Lyc*

storms, of, being alone in   *Phos*

feet *see* **Limbs**

fever   *Acon, Ars, Bell, Euphr, Eup-P, Gels, Nux-V, Puls, Rhus-T*

alternately hot, cold   *Rhus-T*

alternate sides, hot and cold   *Rhus-T*

clammy   *Ars*

chilly   *Gels, Nux-V*

cold food/drink felt instantly in the blood,   *Rhus-T*

during the daytime   *Euphr*

intense   *Acon, Bell*

leading to biliousness/jaundice   *Eup-P*

one-sided   *Rhus-T*

persistent, with chills   *Rhus-T*

restlessness, with   *Eup-P*

thirst, without   *Puls*

fidgety   *Apis Mel*

flatulence   *Arg-N, Ars, Cal-C, Carb-V, Cham, Lyc, Puls, Sil, Sul*

loud   *Arg-N*

foreign bodies, to expel any   *Sil*

forgetful   *Arn, Lyc*

fretful   *Ars, Cham*

frightened   *Acon, Apis Mel, Gels* (*see also* **Fears**)

fussy   *Apis Mel, Ars, Nux-V, Puls*

about appearance   *Sil*

grief   *Acon, Gels, Ign, Nat-M*

inconsolable   *Ign*

suffers in silence   *Nat-M*

suppressed   *Ign, Nat-M*

gums, bleeding   *Ham, Merc*

hair loss, acute, when anaemic   *Phos*

when pregnant   *Sul*

hallucinating, may be violent when   *Bell*

hay fever   *All-C*

head   *Arn, Bell, Calc-C, Carb-V, Cham, Eup-P, Hyp, Ign, Merc, Sul*

blows to   *Arn, Hyp*

cradle cap, sour smelling   *Calc-C*

feels as though clamped in a band   *Merc, Sul*

hot   *Bell, Carb-V, Cham, Merc, Nat-M*

top of, feels   *Sul*

moist   *Cham*

patchy sweating of   *Calc-C*

pierced, feels as though   *Ign*

scalp aches   *Eup-P*

headache   *Acon, All-C, Arg-N,*
   Bell, Bry, Cal-C, Cupr, Euphr,
   Eup-P, Gels, Hep-S, Ign,
   Kali-B, Lyc, Nat-M, Nux-V,
   Phos, Puls, Rhus-T, Ruta, Sil,
   Staph, Sul
   accompanies other symptoms
      Bry
   acute   *Bell, Bry*
   as though bruised and beaten
      Ruta
   back of head   *Eup-P*
      then pain moves to forehead
         or one eye   *Sil*
   bursting   *Eup-P, Euphr*
      affecting sight   *Euphr*
      worse for sweats   *Eup-P*
   catarrhal   *Euphr*
   clamping   *Arg-N, Gels, Merc,*
      Rhus-T, Sul
   congestive   *All-C, Gels*
   disabling   *Calc-C*
   eyes affected
      acute   *Bry*
      over both   *Nux-V, Staph*
      over one   *Phos, Sil*
      sight affected   *Euphr*
   forehead, of, severe   *All-C*
   frontal, affecting eyeballs   *Staph*
   hot   *Nat-M*
   lack of sleep, causes   *Cupr*
   located in small areas   *Kali-B*
   migraine   *Kali-B*
      with vomiting   *Arg-N*
   right sided   *Hep-S*
   tension headaches   *Ign*
   throbbing   *Puls*
      before menstruation, improved
         by cold compress   *Puls*
      dull   *Phos*
      especially when food delayed
         Lyc

rear of head   *Eup-P*
   violent   *Acon*
      when chilled   *Nat-M*
herpes   *Nat-M*
hiccoughs   Carb-V, Nat-M
hives *see* **urticaria**
hormonal disturbances   *Apis*
   Mel, Cal-C, Cupr, Ign, Lyc,
   Merc, Nat-M, Phos, Sep, Sul
hyperactive, especially before
   feared activity   *Arg-N*
hypersensitive to   *Acon, Cal-C,*
   Hep-S, Merc, Nux-V, Phos,
   Sep, Staph
   change   *Merc*
   cold, yet needs fresh air   *Ars*
   criticism   *Calc-C, Staph*
   heat, cold, pain, smell, touch,
      sound, air currents   *Hep-S*
   imagined slights   *Staph*
   loud music   *Sep*
   pain   *Led, Sep, Staph*
   sympathy, rejects all   *Sep*
   temperature extremes   *Sep*
   touch, of infected bites or
      wounds   *Led*
hysterical   *Acon, Bell, Ign, Nat-M,*
   Rhus-T, Sep

imagination, vivid   *Sul*
imagines is ill   *Nux-V*
impatient   *Acon, Cham, Hep-S,*
   Ign, Sul
impulsive   *Arg-N, Hep-S*
inadequacy, **feelings of**, low self-
   esteem   *Lyc*
inconsolable   *Cham, Ign, Nat-M*
indecisive   *Bry, Calc-C, Lyc*
   feigns indifference, to mask
      Calc-C
   helpless due to   *Cal-C*

indignation, for wrongful
   accusation, unexpressed
   Staph
imflammations
   bright red, without discharge
      Acon
   injury site   *Ruta*
   of blood, digestive and
      respiratory systems   *Phos*
   raging   *Canth*
   urinary   *Canth*
influenza *see* **common cold/
   influenza**
injuries (*see also* **cuts and
   lacerations, wounds**)
   where skin broken   *Acon, Cal,
      Hyp*
   where skin unbroken   *Acon,
      Arn, Hyp*
injustice, sense of   *Staph*
insect bites/stings *see* **bites and
   stings**
insomnia   *Ign*
   anxieties, due to   *Lyc*
   early morning   *Nux-V*
   overactive mind, due to   *Puls*
   pain or coughing, due to   *Cham*
   insult, disappointment or
      humiliation, feeling of   *Staph*
intermittent symptoms   *Cupr,
   Ign*
intolerant   *Ign*
introverted *see* **withdrawn**
irritable   *Apis Mel, Arg-N, Arn,
   Bry, Cham, Hep-S, Ign, Ip,
   Lyc, Phos, Puls, Rhus-T,
   Ruta, Sep, Sul*
   on trying to please others   *Phos*
   on waking   *Lyc*
   with depression   *Sep*
   with night terrors   *Rhus-T*

jealous   *Apis Mel, Puls*
joints   *Acon, Kali-B, Led, Puls,
   Rhus-T, Ruta*
   pain in   *Kali-B, Led, Puls,
      Rhus-T, Ruta*
      better for compresses   *Puls*
      which alternates with catarrh
         and diarrhoea   *Kali-B*
   stiff   *Rhus-T*
   swollen   *Led, Rhus-T*
   weak   *Acon*
      after injury healed   *Ruta*
jumpy   *Sil*

labour, after *see* **childbirth**
lazy and quarrelsome   *Sul*
libido, low   *Sep*
lice   *Staph*
limbs
   aching   *Dros*
   feet   *Sep, Sil, Sul*
      cold   *Sep*
      hot, especially at night   *Sul*
      sweaty   *Sil*
   legs and feet cold   *Calc-C, Sep*
   weakened, feel bruised or numb
      Rhus-T
lips   *Ars, Cupr, Hep-S, Nat-M, Sul*
   blue   *Cupr*
   cracked, lower   *Hep-S*
   dry   *Ars, Nat-M*
   red   *Sul*
mania   *Bell, Canth*
mastitis   *Sil*
memory loss   *Arg-N, Carb-V,
   Hyp, Lyc*
   and depression   *Hyp*
   from mental exhaustion/anxiety
      Arg-N, Lyc
   short-term   *Carb-V*
menstruation
   menorrhagia (heavy bleeding)
      and hot flushes   *Phos, Sul*

mental state *see* **individual symptoms**
metabolism *see* **digestion**
methodical and controlling *Bry*
modalities – better for (>)
  activity *Sep*
  alcohol consumption *Gels*
  affection *Phos*
  bedcovers, covering *Nux-V*
    uncovered *Acon, Apis Mel*
  belching *Arg-N, Carb-V*
  clothing, loose *Lyc*
  cold *All-C, Apis Mel, Arg-N, Canth, Led, Puls, Rhus-T*
    applications *Apis Mel, Canth, Led*
    cool room *All-C*
    of any kind, touch, air, weather, etc *Rhus-T*
    shower/bath *Arg-N, Led*
    even if feeling cold *Puls*
  company *Arg-N, Ars*
  consoled, being *Puls*
  deep breath *Ign*
  defecating *Nux-V*
  declining to oblige favours *Staph*
  dry conditions *Cal-C, Sul*
  drinks, for *Arg-N, Ars, Bell, Cupr, Hep-S, Ign, Ip, Lyc, Phos*
    cold *Arg-N, Bell, Cupr, Ip, Phos*
    during the chill *Eup-P*
    hot *Ars, Hep-S, Lyc*
  eating *Ign, Phos, Puls, Sep, Staph*
    breakfast *Staph*
    cold food *Phos, Puls*
  eyes, bathed *Euphr*
    closed *Bry*
  evenings *Nux-V*
  exercise, despite lethargy *Sep*

  flatulence *Lyc, Nux-V*
  fresh air *Acon, All-C, Arg-N, Arn, Carb-V, Dros, Ip, Lyc, Nat-M, Puls, Sep, Sul*
  heat *Ars, Calc-C, Canth, Gels, Hep-S, Ign, Kali-B, Lyc, Nux-V, Rhus-T, Ruta, Sep, Sil, Staph*
    especially applied to the head *Sil*
    (but worse for head symptoms *Ars, Lyc*)
    local application of, for colic *Cham*
    moderate *Gels*
    of any kind, bath, friction *Rhus-T*
  lying down *Arn, Ars, Bry, Calc-C, Euphr, Gels, Ham, Merc, Rhus-T, Ruta*
    on affected side *Bry*
    on back *Ruta*
    on firm surface *Rhus-T*
    on stomach *Merc*
    when constipated *Calc-C*
    yet moves restlessly *Ars*
  massage of pain sites *Phos*
  morning *Merc*
  movement *Cham, Eup-P, Kali-B, Lyc, Puls, Rhus-T, Ruta, Sul*
    after intially worse *Rhus-T*
    gentle *Puls, Ruta*
    infant carried or transported *Cham*
    rocking of infant *Cham*
  position, changes of *Arn, Cham*
    doubled up *Cham*
    knees raised towards chest *Cham*
  pressure *Bry, Cupr, Dros, Gels, Kali-B, Nat-M*

congested area   *Gels*
headache or sinus pain
  Kali-B, Nat-M
holding/binding affected part
  Bry
holding chest while coughing
  Dros
if spasms   *Cupr*
rest   *Bell, Bry, Canth, Cupr,*
  Ham, Hyp, Kali-B, Nat-M,
  Nux-V, Staph
  on affected side   *Hyp*
  undisturbed   *Bry, Ham, (see*
    also, **modalities, better**
    for, sleep)
silence   *Sep*
sitting erect   *Ip, Sep*
sleep   *Nat-M, Nux-V, Phos, Sep*
  short naps, *Sul (see also*
  modalities, better for, rest)
solitude   *Nat-M, Sep*
stimulation, absence of any   *Bell*
sweating   *Cupr, Eup-P* (except
  headache which made worse
  for), *Gels, Nat-M, Rhus-T*
  if not chilled by   *Rhus-T*
tidy surroundings   *Ars*
urinating   *Gels, Lyc, Sil*
walk in fresh air, warmly
  dressed   *Rhus-T, Sep*
warmth   *see* **modalities, better**
  for, heat
water on face, cold splashing
  Phos
weather
  cold air   *Eup-P*
  damp   *Nux-V*
  dry   *Bry, Calc, Sul*
  fresh air   *Acon, All-C, Arg-*
    N, Arn, Carb-V, Dros, Ip,
    Lyc, Nat-M, Puls, Sep, Sul.
  sunshine   *Sep*

warm   *Ars, Calc-C, Canth,*
  Hep-S, Ign, Kali-B, Nux-V,
  Phos, Rhus-T, Ruta, Sep,
  Sil, Staph, Sul
wet   *Hep-S*
mosalities – worse for (<)
alcohol   *Ars*
airless rooms   *Sul*
anger   *Nux-V*
attention   *Cham*
bathing   *Sul*
bedcovers   *Acon, Led, Puls*
  even though feels cool   *Led*
  off *see* **modalities, worse,**
    uncovered
bending, if throbbing headache
  Bell
breathing, cough   *Kali-B*
bright light   *Acon, All-C*
  (headache)
change   *Merc*
clothing; tight, restrictive
  Hep-S, Lyc
comfort   *Sil*
coughing (if chest painful)   *Dros*
demands of others upon self
  Sep
diarrhoea after midday   *Calc-C*
discharges suppressed   *Cupr*
draughts   *Cham, Hep-S, Nat-M,*
  Ruta
drinking   *Ars, Canth, Cham,*
  Dros, Ham, Ign, Led, Lyc,
  Staph
  alcohol, though craves it   *Led*
  chamomile tea   *Cham*
  coffee   *Cham, Ign*
  cold   *Ars, Lyc, Staph*
  despite thirst   *Canth*
  water   *Ham*
eating   *Lyc, Nux-V, Sil, Staph*
  before an event   *Lyc*

irregularly   *Sil, Staph*
effort, physical or mental
   Calc-C, Nux-V, Ruta
emotional arousal   *Phos, Puls,*
   Staph
   negative outbursts   *Staph*
   suppression of   *Puls*
evening   *All-C, Cupr, Phos*
exercise   *Nat-M, Ruta*
   after joint injury healed   *Ruta*
exposure to cold or wet   *Sep*
food   *Arg-N, Arn, Ars, Carb-V,*
   Ign, Ip, Lyc, Puls
   brassicas   *Lyc*
   breads   *Lyc*
   cold   *Arn, Lyc*
   fatty, rich   *Ip, Puls*
   greasy   *Carb-V*
   legumes   *Lyc*
   milk   *Lyc*
   pastries   *Lyc*
   shellfish   *Lyc*
   smell of food   *Ip*
   sweet foods and candies
      Arg-N, Ign
fresh air   *Ham, Hep-S, Ign*
   lack of   *Bry, Puls*
heat   *Arg-N, Bell, Bry, Cham,*
   Nat-M, Puls
   but not better for cold   *Cham*
hunger   *Sep*
light   *Bell, Euphr, Phos, Sil*
lying down   *Dros*
   on affected part   *Ruta*
   on affected side   *Hep-S*
   on left side   *Phos*
   on right side   *Merc*
menstruation   *Calc-C, Cupr,*
   Nat-M, Sep
   delayed   *Sep*
   imminent   *Cupr*
   with PMT   *Nat-M*

movement   *Bell, Bry, Dros,*
   (*Gels* for headache), *Hep-S,*
   Hyp, (*Kali-B* for headache),
   Led, Rhus-T
initially worse for, then better
   for then worse   *Rhus-T*
of injured site with puncture
   wound   *Led*
noise   *Bell, Sep, Sil*
observation   *Calc-C*
overheated, being   *Nat-M*
pressure, applied   *Hyp, Lyc,*
   Ruta, Staph
reclining, cough worse for
   Euphr
rest   *Puls, Sep*
scratching, rash worse for
   Rhus-T
sleep
   being disturbed   *Nux-V*
   nap, mid afternoon   *Staph*
smells   *Bell, Phos*
solitude   *Arg-N, Ars*
standing   *Calc-C, Sep, Sul*
stimulants   *Nux-V*
sweating, if throbbing headache
   at back of head   *Eup-P*
sympathy when upset   *Nat-M*
talking   *Dros*
teething   *Calc-C*
temperature changes   *Ars, Bell,*
   Merc, Phos
   room temperature, changes of
      Phos
   sudden   *Bell*
time
   day time, cough worse for
      Euphr
   early morning, 2–3 am
      Kali-B, Sul
   evening   *Euphr, Phos*
   late morning   *Nat-M*

mid-afternoon *Bell*

midnight, after *Dros*

morning (for digestive upsets) *Puls*

night *Acon, All-C, Ars, Bell, Cham, Cupr, Euphr, Ip, Led, Merc, Nux-V, Rhus-T, Sep, Sul*

sinuses, blocked, worse at *Nux-V*

tobacco smoke, inhaled *Ign, Ip, Staph*

touch *Arn, Bell, Canth, Cham, Cupr, Ham, Hyp, Ign, Phos, Sep, Staph*

of bruises or source of bleeding *Ham, Staph*

uncovered *Sil*

rapidly worsens symptoms *Hep-S*

vomiting *Cupr*

waking *Lyc, Nux-V*

warm room *Acon, Gels, Led, Puls*

warmth *Acon, All-C, Apis Mel, (Ars for headache), Carb-V, Dros, Euphr, Gels, Ip, Led, Puls, Sul*

weather

changeable *Kali-B, Phos*

cold *All-C, Ars, Calc-C, Cham, Euph, Hyp, Ip, Kali-B, Nux-V, Rhus-T, Ruta, Sep, Sil, Staph*

damp *All-C, Calc-C, Sep*

hot *Cupr, Euphr*

humidity *Ip*

sunlight *Cupr, Euphr*

wet *Ars, Cham, Kali-B, Ruta*

wind *Acon, Cham, Euphr, Hep-S, Ruta*

winter *Sil*

moodswings *Apis Mel, Cupr, Ign, Lyc, Merc*

desires company/wants solitude *Phos*

mouth *see* **face**

muscular *Arn, Cupr, Hyp, Led, Ruta*

cramps *Cupr*

injuries failed to heal after acute treatment *Hyp, Led, Ruta*

soreness, aching after exertion/ injury *Arn*

spasms *Cupr, Ign*

sprains/strains *Arn, Led, Ruta*

stiffness, pain, difficulty getting up *Rhus-T*

better for movement after initially worse *Rhus-T*

tone, slack *Sep*

twitches *Ign*

nail beds, crushed/torn *Hyp*

nausea *Acon, Cupr, Eup-P, Ip, Nat-M, Nux-V*

accompanies any other symptoms *Ip*

after a chill *Eup-P*

after exposure to sun *Nat-M*

sudden *Acon*

without vomiting, unable to vomit *Nux-V*

nervous system

bites affecting nerves *Hyp*

disrupted *Bell*

jerking *Bell*

rapid movements and speech *Arg-N*

seizure *Cupr*

trembling *Arg-N*

twitching *Bell, Cupr*

wounds involving neural pathways *Hyp*

nettle rash *see* **Urticaria**

nightmares see **Dreams**
nipples
cracked, *Cal* (remove cream or
tincture before breastfeeding)
nose *All-C, Hep-S, Ip, Phos*
congested with a cold *Ip*
discharge from *All-C*
one side blocked, swollen; thin
bloody mucus from other
Phos
pains at base of right side of
Hep-S
nosebleed
frequent *Puls*
persistent *Ham*
ulcerated *Sil*
nurses grievances, guilt and hurt
feelings *Nat-M*

obese *Calc-C, Nux-V*
obsessionally tidy *Arn, Ars,
Nux-V*
offence, easily takes *Calc-C,
Cham, Dros, Staph*
onset
over a few hours *Ip*
right-sided *Apis Mel*
slow *Gels, Kali-B, Lyc*
over several days *Bry*
sudden *Acon, Apis Mel, Ars,
Hep-S, Ip*
after exposure to cold wind
Bell
and violent *Bell*
burning pains *Canth*
traumatic *Arn*
overindulgence see **excess**
oversensitive *Arn, Ars, Bell,
Cham, Staph*
to cold yets needs fresh air *Ars*
to pain or being touched *Arn,
Cham, Staph*
overwork see **excess**

pains, nature and location of
aching *Rhus-T*
acute *Acon, Cham, Hyp, Kali-B*
concentrated in small area(s)
of a few centimetres *Kali-B*
unbearable, cries out *Cham*
worse for movement *Hyp*
ascend spine from lower back
Hyp
back *Kali-B, Nat-M, Nux-V,
Phos, Puls, Rhus-T*
after exposure to draughts
Nux-V
after effort *Nat-M*
and sprains *Puls*
base of spine *Kali-B*
after effort *Nat-M*
lower back *Nat-M, Puls*
rheumaticky, aching in
Rhus-T
shoulder blades, between
Kali-B
bites, stings, puncture wounds,
painful to the touch *Led*
bones, aching (or as if) *Eup-P*
brief *Acon*
burning *Acon, Apis Mel, Arn,
Ars, Canth, Phos, Sul*
but better for heat *Ars*
changeable, rapidly *Kali-B*
colicky, with diarrhoea *Cham*
dragging, dull, aching *Sep*
earache, very sensitive to cold
air *Cham, Hep-S*
worse on left side *Kali-B*
fierce *Acon*
front through to back of chest
Kali-B
glands, burning, searing pains
in *Phos*
intense *Acon, Cham, Hyp,
Kali-B*

intermittent, in different places
  Kali-B
itching *Sul*
joints and ligaments, in *Rhus-T*
mouth, sore around, after
  exposure to sun *Nat-M*
pelvis, downward pressure on
  as if bruised *Sep*
  post-operative pains and
    infections *Staph*
right-sided, may cross to left
  later, or from above to below
  Lyc
scalding *Canth*
searing, sharp *Hep-S, Hyp,
  Phos, Rhus-T*
sexual system, post-operative,
  pain *Staph*
shooting *Bell, Hyp, Nat-M*
  along nerve path *Hyp*
soreness
  as if bones were broken
    Eup-P
spasmodic *Bell*
splintering *Arg-N, Hep-S*
stinging *Acon, Apis Mel*
stitching, shooting *Nat-M*
throbbng *Bell*
thumping, on top of head *Nux-V*
unbearable *Cham*
urinary, post-operative *Staph*
wandering *Led*
wound site *Ruta*
panics *Acon*
perspiration *see* **sweat**
posture *see* **appearance**
**precipitating conditions, recent
    case of...**
  accidents *Arn, Hyp*
  aged, infirm and weak *Carb-V*
  allergic reaction *All-C, Apis
    Mel*

assault *Staph*
bathing *Sul*
bites and stings (insect) *Apis
  Mel, Arn, Canth, Hyp, Led*
  shooting pains, caused by
    Hyp
  which punctured *Led*
blow to eye area, bruising from
  Led
burns *Canth*
carbon monoxide poisoning
  Carb-V
chamomile tea, drunk to excess
  Cham
change, of diet, temperature,
  water, etc. *Merc*
children, demands of, overtire
  mother *Sep*
childbirth *Acon, Arn, Cal,
    Cham, Cupr, Gels, Ham,
    Hyp, Puls, Ruta, Sep, Staph*
  cramps after *Cupr*
  episiotomy *Hyp*
  forceps or caesarian delivery
    Arn, Cal, Hyp, Staph
  haemorrhoids after *Ham*
  post natal problems *Sep*
colds, influenza, fevers *Acon,
    Bry, Eup-P, Euphr, Hep-S,
    Merc, Nux-V, Phos, Puls,
    Rhus-T, Sep*
colic *Cham*
croup in childhood *Hep-S*
cuts and wounds *see* injuries
death, a, *see* emotions,
  bereavement
dental treatment *Cal, Phos*
ear infection, prior *Puls*
efforts which caused sweat and
  chill *Bry*
emotions *Apis Mel, Bell,
    Cham, Gels, Ip, Puls, Staph*

anger   *Cham, Ip, Staph*
  raving   *Bell*
  suppressed   *Staph*
anxiety, financial   *Bry, Gels,
  Ign, Lyc*
bereavement   *Acon, Gels,
  Ign, Nat-M, Puls, Staph*
disappointment, acute   *Ign,
  Staph*
fear   *Acon, Arg-N, Gels, Ign,
  Lyc*
  fright   *Acon, Ign*
  pre-examination nerves
    Arg-N, Gels, Ign, Lyc
grief *see* bereavement
heartbroken   *Ign*
homesick   *Ign*
indignation   *Staph*
jealousy, intense   *Ign*
love affair, failed   *Ign, Nat-M,
  Staph*
panic   *Acon*
rejection or reprimand   *Nat-M*
shame or embarrassment   *Gels*
shock   *Acon, Carb-V, Gels,
  Ign*
  especially with trembling
    Gels
  suppression of   *Ign*
stage fright   *Arg-N, Ign*
excess, of any kind   *Nux-V*
  coffee, too much   *Cham*
  of cold   *Sul*
  of eating   *Ip, Sul*
  of effort or exercise   *Sul*
  of heat   *Sul*
  overwork   *Arn, Nux-V, Rhus-T,
    Ruta, Sul*
  physical exertion has brought
    on a chill   *Ars*
  exposure to draught, which led
    to back pain   *Nux-V*

eye conditions, prior   *Euphr, Puls*
fair-skinned person   *Phos*
food poisoning   *Ars*
fractures   *Ruta*
hangover   *Kali-B, Nux-V*
haemorrahge after injury/dental
  extraction   *Ham, Phos*
hay fever   *Euphr*
head cold   *Euphr*
injuries   *Acon, Arn, Cal, Carb-V,
  Hyp, Led, Rhus-T, Ruta*
  affecting nerve-rich areas   *Hyp*
  crushed finger/thumb/toe ends
    Hyp
  joints, ligaments   *Led, Ruta*
  lower back injury   *Hyp*
  puncture wounds   *Hyp, Led,
    Staph*
labour, pains of *see* childbirth
lice   *Staph*
measles, incompletely recovered
  from   *Carb-V, Puls*
menopause   *Cupr, Phos, Sep,
  Sul*
menses, delayed   *Cupr, Sep*
mental effort, intense   *Arg-N*
nerve-related problems   *Hyp*
mumps, swollen glands   *Rhus-T,
  Ruta, Sul*
overheated environment   *Acon,
  Bell, Bry, Gels, Nat-M, Puls*
oxygen starvation (until help
  arrives)   *Carb-V*
pregnancy
  baby high in womb   *Carb-V*
  nausea in   *Ip*
pre-menstrual tension   *Cupr,
  Nat-M*
red-haired person   *Phos*
sleep disturbed   *Nux-V*
splinter in skin   *Hyp*
suppression of

cold symptoms leading to
  headache   *Calc-C*
emotions   *Ip*
surgery, following   *Hyp, Rhus-T,*
  Staph
  lumbar puncture   *Hyp*
  surgical interventions, using
    sharp implements   *Staph*
  when nerves sore   *Hyp*
toothache   *Cal, Phos, Staph*
  teething infant   *Cham, Cupr,*
  Puls
temperature changes, recent
  Merc
tuberculosis, family history of
  Dros
urinary infections   *Canth*
victim   *Staph*
waking, on   *Lyc*
weather
  changeable   *Kali-B, Merc,*
    Rhus-T, Sul
    especially cold to warm
      Bry, Gels, Sul
    season changes   *Bry, Kali-B*
  cold   *Acon, Calc-C, Kali-B,*
    Rhus-T, Sil
  cold wind, exposure to   *All-C,*
    Bell, Hep-S, Nux-V, Rhus-T
  damp   *All-C, Calc-C, Sil*
  dry wind   *Acon, Hep-S*
  electrical storms   *Phos*
  over-exposure to sun   *Acon,*
    Bry, Canth, Nat-M, Puls
  wet, exposure to, especially
    Rhus-T
    the head   *Bell*
    the feet   *Puls, Rhus-T, Sil*
whooping cough   *Dros*
  incompletely recovered from
    Carb-V
pulse, fast   *Bell*

pus *see* **discharges**

rash *see* **skin**
raving   *Bell*
respiration   *All-C, Ars, Bry, Eup-P,*
  Hep-S, Ip, Lyc, Nux-V, Phos
  bronchitis   *Phos*
    with nausea   *Ip*
  chest, tight, painful   *All-C,*
    Eup-P, Nux-V
    worse for coughing   *Phos*
  choking   *Ip*
  cough with nausea   *Ip*
  difficult   *Ars, Eup-P, Ip*
    sits with hands on knees to
      ease   *Eup-P*
    shoulders raised, to ease
      Eup-P
  infection, chest   *Bry*
  laboured   *Eup-P*
  mouth breathing, when nasally
    congested   *Lyc*
  rapid   *Ip*
  wheezy   *Ars, Hep-S, Ip*
restless   *Acon, Arg-N, Ars, Bell,*
  Canth, Dros, Eup-P, Lyc,
  Merc, Puls, Rhus-T, Ruta
  to escape pain, though wishes
    to be still   *Eup-P*
retching   *Nux-V*
ridicule, deeply unsettled by   *Nat-M*

sad   *Apis Mel, Ign, Sep*
saliva, absent   *Nat-M*
sandals, usually worn in all
  weathers   *Sul*
scalds *see* **burns and scalds**
scornful of others   *Ip*
selfish   *Sul*
  oblivious of needs of others
    when ill, cares for when well
    Sep
self-assured   *Nat-M*

self doubting *Ruta*
  fears exposure *Lyc*
self pitying *Led, Puls*
sensations *see also* **Pain**
  chilly *Eup-P*
    but desires cold rooms and
      drinks *Phos*
  heat rises up back or chest
    Phos
  heaviness *Gels*
  numbness *Cham*
  stinging, burning *Apis Mel,
    Canth*
  throbbing *Bell*
senses
  all heightened *Bell, Hep-S,
    Nux-V*
  disturbed *Gels*
  mentally dull, only when ill
    Phos
  photosensitive *Euphr, Merc*
  roaring sounds *Ign*
  touch, angers *Hep-S*
  vision
    affected by local bruising
      Ham
    blurred *Gels*
sensitive *see* **hypersensitive**
shaking *see* **trembling**
shirks responsibility, yet very
  good worker *Sil*
shivers *Eup-P*
shock *Acon, Apis Mel, Arn, Hyp*
  following injury to nerves
    Hyp
shoulders, raised *see* **appearance**
shy *Lyc, Nat-M, Puls*
  when urinating *Nat-M*
  when weeping *Nat-M*
sided symptoms
    alternate sides are hot and cold
      Rhus-T

  one *Puls, Rhus-T*
  right *Apis Mel, Bell, Canth,
    Hep-S*
    headache *Hep-S*
    pains, may cross to left later,
      or from above to below *Lyc*
  left *Sep*
    earache worse on *Kali-B*
    lies on, when *Phos*
sighs, large *Ign*
silent *Merc*
  brooding *Ign*
  tears *Ign*
sinus problems *Kali-B, Lyc,
  Nux-V*
skin *Acon, All-C, Apis Mel, Bell,
  Cal, Canth, Cupr, Gels, Hep-
  S, Hyp, Nat-M, Rhus-T, Sil,
  Sul*
  blotchy *Gels*
  boils, spots, pimples, slow to
    heal *Hep-S*
  burnt or scalded *Canth*
  cold to the touch *Arn, Calc-C*
  cuts, abrasions *Cal*
  dry *Acon, Nat-M, Sul*
    hot, without sweat *Acon,
      Nat-M*
    scaly *Sul*
  hot to the touch *Apis Mel,
    Bell*
  infections of, suppurating
    Hep-S
  rash *Apis Mel, Cal, Rhus-T*
    after exposure to wet *Rhus-T*
    incomplete or slow to appear
      Apis Mel
    itchy, red heat rash under the
      skin *Rhus-T*
    nappy/diaper *Cal*
    raised, rough to touch *Apis
      Mel*

scars, pain from   *Hyp*
sores, upper lip and around
     nose   *All-C*
splinter   *Sil*
     painful and inflamed   *Hyp*
spots, pimples and ulcers, itchy
     Cupr
sunburn   *Canth*
sleep
disturned pattern of   *Nux-V*
great desire to   *Eup-P*
lack of   *Nux-V*
nightmares   *Ign, Nat-M*
profound, with twitching
     spasms   *Cupr*
sleepwalking   *Ign*
sneezing   *Eup-P, Euphr*
forceful on breathing cold air
     All-C
frequent   *All-C*
rising from rest, on   *All-C*
sudden fit of   *Acon*
soreness *see* **pains**
spasms   *Ign*
cramping, alternates with
     exhaustion   *Cupr*
painful, start at extremities   *Cupr*
painful, move upwards   *Cupr*
spiteful   *Nux-V*
splinters   *Hyp, Sil*
sprains/strains *see* **muscular**
stings *see* **bites and stings**
stomach
bloated and gaseous   *Carb-V*
cramps, violent   *Cupr*
distended   *Arg-N*
pains   *Staph*
stools
blood streaked, though pain free
     Phos
difficulty in passing, retracts
     when partly emerged   *Sil*

foul smelling   *Merc, Sul*
frequent yet incomplete   *Nux-V*
green   *Ip, Merc*
small, dry, pellets   *Nat-M*
stubborn, yet indecisive and shy
     Calc-C
stupefied   *Bry*
sullen   *Bry*
sunburn *see* **skin**
sunstroke   *Bell, Nat-M*
suppressed emotions   *Ign, Nat-M*
surgery
before   *Arn*
following   *Arn, Staph*
stretching or cutting of tissues,
     surgical, traumatic   *Staph*
suspicious, of others' motives   *Dros*
feels victimised and cheated
     Dros
sweats   *Calc-C, Staph*
active or resting, if   *Rhus-T*
at night   *Hep-S*
cold   *Acon, Ars, Ip, Sep*
     but needs fanning   *Carb-V*
covering produces   *Bell*
easily   *Rhus-T, Sep, Sul*
frequent, of body, not head
     Rhus-T
exertion, after, leading to a chill
     Rhus-T
     after minimal   *Calc-C*
hot   *Ip, Nux-V, Sep*
localized   *Puls*
offensive   *Hep-S, Puls, Sep, Sul*
sour   *Lyc*
patchy   *Sep*
     especially of head   *Calc-C*
profuse   *Sul*
     although patient is not hot
          Merc
     especially at night, of head,
          hands and feet   *Sil*

scanty *Eup-P*
suppressed *Sil*
swelling *Apis Mel, Arn, Calc-C,*
Hep-S, Kali-B, Merc, Ruta,
Sil, Staph, Sul
abdomen, of *Sul*
after dental/surgical treatment
Arn
fibrous, at site of overexertion
Ruta
glands *Calc-C, Hep-S, Merc,*
Sil, Sul
hard to the touch *Calc-C*
local *Ruta*
prostate *Staph*
puffiness *Apis Mel*
shiny red, itchy *Apis Mel*
testes, from mumps *Staph*
tonsils *Kali-B*
swollen *see* **swelling**

tantrums, childish *Ip*
taste
awakes with bad *Puls*
bitter, with dry lips/mouth
Ars, Nat-M
metallic *Cupr, Merc, Rhus-T*
unpleasant *Sul*
tearful *Carb-V, Cham, Ign, Nat-*
M, Phos, Puls, Rhus-T, Ruta,
Sep
in solitude *Nat-M*
sobs silently *Ign*
suppressed unless alone *Nat-M*
when ill *Sep*
teeth, concerning
abscesses beneath *Sil*
after dental treatment *Arn,*
Cal
teething pains *Cham*
temperamental *Cham, Cupr*
hard to please *Nux-V*

temperature
high *Acon*
high without thirst *Apis Mel*
sudden drop in *Acon*
tendons, injured *Led*
theological/philosophical/religious
passions *Sul*
thirst *Apis Mel, Gels, Ign, Nux-V,*
Puls, Rhus-T, Sil
absence of *Apis Mel, Gels,*
Nux-V, Puls
when feels hot *Ign*
acute, yet difficulty swallowing
Rhus-T
for cold drinks *Arg-N, Bry,*
Cham, Eup-P, Led, Merc,
Ruta
great *Acon, Bry, Nat-M, Ruta*
great, yet wants infrequent
small sips *Ars*
water, for *Sul*
when feels cold *Ign*
yet craves salt *Nat-M*
throat *Acon, All-C, Arg-N, Ars,*
Bell, Dros, Hep-S, Ign, Kali-
B, Merc, Nux-V, Phos, Rhus-T
dry *Ars, Bell*
inflamed, severely *Kali-B*
larynx and throat glands,
swollen and sore *Rhus-T*
lump in, as if, eased by eating
Ign
persistent tickle *All-C, Dros*
sharp pains *All-C, Arg-N,*
Hep-S, Nux-V
sore *Merc, Phos*
after exposure to dry, cold
wind *Acon*
begins on right side *Lyc*
swallowing difficult *Calc-C,*
Canth, Dros, Merc, Nux-V
swollen *Merc*

splintered   *Hep-S, Nux-V*

time-affected
diarrhoea, urgent, early morning
   Sul
fever during the day   *Euphr*
hunger, midmorning   *Sul*
sweats at night   *Hep-S*
symptoms
   begin at night, commonly
      Rhus-T
   come and go   *Bell, Cham*
      at regular times   *Kali-B*
   worse at set times, various   *Lyc*
   4am   *Nux-V*
   4am and 8am   *Lyc*
timid *see* **shy**
tiredness *see* **exhaustion**
tongue   *Merc, Nat-M, Puls,*
   Rhus-T, Sul
   blistered   *Nat-M*
   furred   *Merc, Puls, Rhus-T, Sul*
   red-tipped and sore   *Rhus-T*
   yellow or white coating   *Kali-B,*
   Merc, Puls, Rhus-T
   white, with red tip and edges
      Sul
tonsils *see entry* for symptom, e.g.
   swelling
torpid   *Calc-C*
trauma *see* **injuries**
travel sickness   *Staph*
trembling, shaking   *Gels, Ign,*
   Staph

ulcers   *Cupr, Kali-B, Merc, Sil*
   mucous membranes ulcerated
      Kali-B, Merc
unassertive, outwardly, with inner
   resilience   *Sil*
unexpressed feelings, humiliation,
   anger, indignation   *Staph*
urination

burns on   *Canth, Staph*
blood in   *Canth*
frequent   *Gels, Nux-V, Staph*
   to little effect   *Canth*
foul smelling   *Merc*
scant   *Apis Mel*
shy about at any age   *Nat-M*
stress incontinence   *Staph*
urticaria/nettle rash/hives   *Cupr*

vaccination, negative reaction to
   Sil
vague   *Nat-M*
veins
   congested   *Ham*
   family history of varicosed   *Ham*
   varicosed   *Calc-C, Ham*
vertigo   *Arg-N, Cupr*
vision, disturbed   *Gels, Kali-B*
   with headache   *Nat-M* (**seek**
      urgent medical help)
vitality, lacks   *Carb-V, Kali-B,*
   Merc, Phos, Sep (*see also*
   exhaustion)
voice   *Arg-N, Ars, Dros, Hep-S,*
   Lyc, Phos
   hoarse   *Ars, Dros, Hep-S*
   loss of   *Phos*
      when anxious   *Arg-N*
   screams on waking   *Lyc*
      while asleep   *Lyc*
   speaks rapidly   *Hep-S*
vomiting   *Acon, Arg-N, Ars,*
   Calc-C, Cupr, Eup-P, Ip,
   Nat-M, Nux-V, Phos
   after a chill   *Eup-P*
   after cold food or drink   *Phos*
   after exposure to sun   *Nat-M*
   after warm drink   *Phos*
   green   *Ip*
   impossible though nauseous
      Nux-V

with diarrhoea, offensive   *Ars*
with migraine   *Arg-N*
with other complaints   *Ip*
sudden   *Acon*
warmth, rejects all kinds of,
  though chilly   *Puls*
weakness   *Calc-C, Lyc, Ruta*
disproportionate to symptoms
  Ars
of joints   *Acon*
weeping *see* **Tearful**
whiny   *Puls*
withdrawn   *Gels, Ign, Merc,
  Nat-M*
and sad   *Ign, Merc*
rejects all change including care
  Merc
suppresses emotions   *Nat-M*

whooping cough (pertussis) *see*
  cough
wilful; child has tantrums but is
  impossible to please   *Ip*
wind *see* **flatulence**
worried   *Arg-N, Ars*
worse for... *see* **modalities –
  worse for**
wounds   *Acon, Arn, Cal, Hyp*
puncture   *Hyp, Led*
stab   *Staph*
suppurating   *Hep-S*
which involve damage to
  nerves   *Hyp*

yawns   frequently   *Ig*

11 | THE MATERIA MEDICA – THE DRUG PICTURES

What is the Materia Medica? As the Latin name might suggest, the name can be translated as Medical Material. Arranged according to symptoms, mental, emotional and physical from head to toe, each entry is a full description of the results of provings. The practical application of these remedies over time has led to a continuing process of personal verification by the homeopaths who have prescribed the remedies and a constant refining of the Materia Medica. There are thus many versions of Materia Medica available. As mentioned, proving involves the careful noting of the symptoms which a homeopathically prepared substance produces in a healthy volunteer, in the assumption that if the same remedy is taken by a sick person experiencing these symptoms, it will trigger a curative reaction. The homeopathic Materia Medica is a list of the results of such provings by healthy volunteers, from the earliest provings by Hahnemann and his followers, to those tested by volunteers today. (Materia Medica do exist for allopathic medicines too, though they describe the effects of the listed drugs upon a sick person, and are intended for use on a broad spectrum of people considered to have the same disease. Any homeopathic Materia Medica describes the symptoms produced in a well person who takes the remedy and thereby indicates the symptoms it will cure in an individual sick person with those same symptoms.) The homeopath seeking the correct remedy for a patient relies upon information recorded in the Materia Medica to match the symptoms presented by a patient with the most suitable remedy as it would be impossible to remember them all.

You will find a simplified Materia Medica and Repertory of Symptoms in this book. It is limited to the remedies most likely and suitable for the first aid this book is intended to address. If, however, the symptom picture you are seeking is not matched within this list you should assume that the condition presented to you ought to be referred to a professional homeopath, since it is beyond the scope recommended for amateur prescribing. This is especially true for chronic, longterm illness, or when a remedy has not effected a cure but instead has aggravated symptoms which did not quickly clear up. Help must also be sought from a professional if you accidentally trigger a proving response. This, you will remember, is the appearance of new symptoms known to be associated with the remedy taken which were not present before. A professional homeopath will have stronger remedies and the experience of prescribing to correct such problems.

The Materia Medica used by professional homeopaths is so large that it cannot be reproduced here. This is a limited list of homeopathic remedies, selected for most common home use and first aid. Do bear in mind that every case is individual and unique, and well-observed symptoms may dictate a remedy other than those suggested here. Beware of forcing a remedy selection by choosing to ignore a peculiar symptom which differs from the proved remedy, although it seems such a good match otherwise. It may be this very exception which indicates a different remedy altogether, perhaps one beyond the scope of this list. Remember it is the odd characteristics by which we distinguish one face from another, when everyone has the same basic features. As a generality, such defining peculiarities will be obvious, rather than slight.

Aconite (Aconitum Napellus)

Usual abbreviation: Aconite or Acon

 Sudden onset   Fright/shock

Thirst for cold drinks   Great fear

Remedy made from Monk's Hood (Wolf's Bane) *Caution: Plant very poisonous to touch or eat in its natural state*

Key words

Onset sudden and fierce but brief; after shock or exposure to cold, dry wind/too much sun; redness, cold sweats; dryness, choking cough; severe pain; weak joints; high fever, great thirst; anxious, fears death.

Possible precipitating situations

Shock; unexpected bereavement, fright or fear of death. Following sudden exposure to cold, too much sun or a dry wind. Birth trauma; sudden accident.

Main signs and symptoms

General/physical

- Sudden onset, pains intense, fierce, brief.
- Red faced, pales with any effort.
- Acute pain.
- Intense fever, dry cough.
- Sudden sneezing fit.
- High temperature.
- Strong thirst, craves cold water to drink.
- Burning, stinging pains cannot bear to be touched.
- Sore throat after exposure to dry, cold wind; sudden drop in temperature.
- Inflammations bright red without discharge, worse on one side.
- Violent headache; sudden vomiting or nausea.
- Skin dry and hot, without sweat.

Mental/emotional

- Restless; agitated, easily startled.
- Panicking, impatient.
- Fearful, anxious, sensitive.

Modalities

Worse: if covered, touched; in bright light; in warm room or in cold winds; at night.

Better: for fresh air if uncovered.

Look for different remedy if . . .

The symptoms are not sudden and intense in nature; the condition lingers, as this remedy is only effective within the first 24–48 hours; behaviour is calm and relaxed; not averse to touch.

Also consider . . .

Arnica; Belladonna; Hepar Sulph; Calcarea Carbonica; and other remedies according to notable symptoms.

Allium (Allium Cepa)

Usual abbreviation: Allium or All-C

 Past exposure cold/damp weather

 Better for fresh air

Worse for warmth

Worse in the evening

Remedy made from red onions.

Key words

Common cold and cough symptoms; hay fever; eyes burn and water; worse for nights/warmth.

Possible precipitating situations

Allergic reactions. Penetrating cold winds, and dampness. Allium Cepa often matches the typical symptoms of a cold unless specific symptoms suggest another remedy.

Main signs and symptoms

General/physical

■ Watery nasal discharge, worse on one side, and frequent sneezing.

■ Nasal discharges burn.

- Sores on upper lip and the skin around the nose caused by discharge
- Persistent tickle in throat, worse in cold air.
- Severe pain in forehead. Congestive headache.
- Sharp pain in throat, as if swallowed razor blades.
- Reluctance to cough for fear of jarring painful throat and headache.
- Tight, painful chest.
- Forceful sneezing on breathing cold air, and on rising from rest.

Mental/emotional

None of note.

Modalities

Worse: in the evening, for damp, cold air, and for warmth. Headache becomes worse in bright light.
Better: in the open air, if not damp; in a cool room.

Look for different remedy if . . .

Onset follows exposure to cold, dry wind. Onset was slow. Little or no sneezing. Cough loose and productive without pain.

Also consider . . .

Aconite; Arsenicum Album; Euphrasia; Gelsemium; Nat Mur; Pulsatilla; and other remedies according to notable symptoms.

Apis Mellifica (Honey bee)

Usual abbreviation: Apis Mel or Apis

 Hot/red swellings   Thirst absent

Better for cold   Worse for touch

Remedy made from the honey bee, complete with venom.

Key words

Stinging, burning pains; no thirst; shiny red swellings following bites, food allergy or stings. Symptoms (often right-sided) which appear after intense, negative emotions.

Possible precipitating situations

Startling, emotionally charged news; a fright, anger or jealousy. A rash which failed to develop fully or is slow to appear. Allergic reactions. Bites or stings which rapidly produce shiny, red swellings that itch.

Main signs and symptoms

General/physical

Stinging, burning sensations. Itchy, red, swellings, puffiness.

Skin rashes are raised and rough. Dislikes skin being touched.

Feels hot to the touch, face reddened, flushed.

Eyelids swollen, eyes watery.

Absence of thirst even though feels hot.

Allergic, histamine reactions to insect bites, stings or food.

Rapid onset and swelling, commencing on right side.

Scant urination.

Mental/emotional

Mood swings.

Fidgety, avoids being touched.

Irritable; fearful; jealous; sad; pernickety.

Cries out in pain.

Modalities

Better: uncovered; for cold applications and for being kept cool.
Worse: for any kind of heat, for touch.

Look for different remedy if . . .

Throbbing rather than stinging or burning. Slow onset. Better for heat. No swelling or redness. Thirsty.

Also consider . . .

Aconitum Napellus; Belladonna; Ledum Palustre; and other remedies according to notable symptoms.

Argent Nit (Argentum Nitricum)

Usual abbreviation: Arg-N

 Anticipatory anxiety

 Better cold; drinks, showers, baths

 Craves, but worse for candy

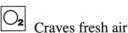 Craves fresh air

Remedy made from pure crystals of silver nitrate (AGNO3) also known as Lunar Caustic and Devil's Stone.

Key words

Dyspepsia, flatulence, diarrhoea; craves sweets, fats, salt. Worried. Performance anxiety. Trembling. Clamping headaches. Impulsive and irritable behaviour.

Possible precipitating situations

Intense mental effort. Stage fright. Pre-performance anxiety, as before public speaking or an exam.

Main signs and symptoms

General/physical

- Anxiety accompanied with trembling and weakness.
- Craving for sugary food, although it produces flatulence and diarrhoea.

- Eye conditions, with discharges.
- Rapid movements and speech.
- Thirst for cold drinks.
- Migraine headaches as though head is clamped, followed by vomiting.
- Disrupted appetite.
- Pains, splinter-like.
- Distended stomach with loud belching and flatulence.
- Irritable bowel; alternate constipation and diarrhoea.
- Loss of voice, especially if anxious about public speaking/singing.
- Throat raw and sharply painful.

Mental/emotional

- Restless, impulsive, hyperactive especially before dreaded activity.
- Fears the outcome of events; fears failure.
- Loss of memory from mental exhaustion and anxiety.
- Claustrophobia; vertigo.
- Afraid of heights and crowded places.

Modalities

Better: for fresh air and the company of others; for belching and flatulence, though it may be difficult to pass wind. Cold drinks. Better for cold shower or bath.

Worse: after eating, especially sugary food or candies; for being alone; for heat.

Look for different remedy if . . .

Paralyzing anxiety before an event, then withdrawn stillness. Quiet fear. No trembling or hyperactivity. Sweets and fatty foods have no ill effects.

Also consider . . .

Gelsemium, Lycopodium; and other remedies according to notable symptoms.

Arnica (Arnica Montana)

Usual abbreviation: Arn

 Fears and is worse for touch

 Better for fresh air

 Hot face; cold extremities

Remedy made from the plant, Leopard's Bane, including its root. Available in the traditional homeopathic format, but also as a cream, ointment or lotion for external use only. NB: Taken internally Arnica helps to arrest bleeding but it should NEVER be applied externally to open cuts/wounds/broken skin.

Key words

Injuries; shock; physical exhaustion; bruises; sprains; hypersensitive to pain and touch; before or after surgical or dental intervention; immediately after bite or sting. Denies is unwell.

Possible precipitating situations

Following trauma, shock, injuries; taken internally for bleeding, cuts, burns, fractures. Especially useful whenever there is swelling and bruising, for example, following surgical or dental treatment; childbirth, fractures, sports injuries, road traffic accident. Immediately after wasp stings. External use only where no broken skin.

Main signs and symptoms

General/physical

■ Sore, bruised and aching especially following exertion or injury.

■ Onset follows trauma.

■ Stress following accident.

■ Hot face, redness, but cold extremities.

■ Cold to the touch.

■ Burning pains.

■ Pale appearance.

Mental/emotional

■ In shock, may deny illness and refuse assistance, even when clearly ill.

■ Fear of medical assistance, of being touched where sore.

■ Angry, irritable, depressed, forgetful.

■ Anxious and obsessionally tidy.

Modalities

Better: for fresh air; for lying down; for changes of position.
Worse: if touched; for food, especially if cold.

Look for different remedy if . . .

Deep internal injuries; injuries to the nervous system. Sprained muscles and joints rather than bruised or cut. Treatment is not given soon after the trauma. Must be no broken skin if applied externally.

Also consider . . .

Aconitum Napellus; Hamamelis; Hypericum; Rhus Toxicodendron; and other remedies according to notable symptoms.

Arsenicum (Arsenicum Album)

Usual abbreviation: Ars

 Burning pains eased by heat

 Feels chilly but pains burn

 Thirst but tolerates only sips

 Restless anxiety

Remedy made from arsenic trioxide, also called white oxide of metallic arsenic. This immutable poisonous base element is rendered safe and homeopathically effective by the process of roasting natural arsenides of iron, nickel and cobalt, followed by trituration and dilution.

Key words

Restlessness; fearful anxiety; burning pains; dry throat; breathing difficulties; weakness disproportionate to symptoms; great thirst yet wants only small sips, infrequently. Food poisoning. Sight and smell of food repels. Made anxious by untidy surroundings.

Possible precipitating situations

When chilled during physical exertion. Food poisoning precipitating burning diarrhoea.

Main signs and symptoms

General/physical

- Burning pains which are better for heat.
- Great exhaustion yet restless; weakness disproportionate to illness.
- Sudden onset of symptoms.
- Vomiting, flatulence and diarrhoea which burns; offensive.
- Thin and watery discharges which burn.
- Face may be hot to the touch yet rest of the body will feel cold.
- Very sensitive and complaining if exposed to cold, yet needs fresh air.
- Easily susceptible to catching colds. Hoarse voice and wheezy chest.
- Dry lips, mouth and bitter taste.
- Craves sips of cold water (cannot tolerate more), may vomit.
- Clammy if has a fever, cold sweats only.
- Appears pale and as if suffering.

Mental/emotional

- Extremely restless, fussy and worried.
- Dislikes untidy environment. Controlling nature.
- Anxiety greater if woken during the night.

- ■ Fears death and loss of control. Doubts will get well again.
- ■ Fretful, critical, angry. Difficult to treat.
- ■ Depressed and afraid of being alone.
- ■ Nightmares and anxiety dreams.

Modalities

Better: if lying down, though moves restlessly; for warmth*; for hot drinks; for tidy surroundings; for company. *The Arsenicum headache (only) is better for cold and cold compresses.
Worse: for cold drinks, alcohol or food, though thirsts for sips of cold water; worse if exposed to temperature changes, cold air or wet weather. At night; alone.

Look for different remedy if . . .

Burning pains not improved by heat. Desires cold (except if has an Arsenicum headache). Desires cold drinks and can tolerate them. Particularly anxious concerning the future. Suffers without complaint.

Also consider . . .

Argenticum Nitricum; Belladonna; Phosphorus; and other remedies according to notable symptoms.

Belladonna (Atropa Belladonna)

Usual abbreviation: Bell

 Thirst cold/lemon drinks

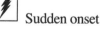 Sudden onset

 Hot, dry fever/red

Delirious/fearful

Remedy made from the Deadly Nightshade (Solanaceae) plant when in flower. *Caution all parts of the plant in its natural state are extremely poisonous.*

Key words

Throbbing; heat; redness. Red faced, red streaks, fast pulse, pupils dilated. Sunstroke. Dry cough/throat. Sudden onset after exposure to cold wind. Symptoms come and go. Delirious; violent temper; hypersensitive.

Possible precipitating situations

Exposure, especially of the head, to cold, dry wind, or to becoming wet.

Main signs and symptoms

General/physical

■ Sudden and violent onset.
■ Shooting, throbbing, spasmodic pains.
■ Fever, violent heat. Hot head.
■ Dry inflammations, dry mucous membranes.
■ Red streaks or rashes.
■ Disrupted nervous system, mental disturbances.
■ Eyes staring and glassy, pupils dilated.
■ Hot to the touch. Sweats where covered.
■ Symptom mainly on the right side of the body.
■ Extremities cold.
■ Symptoms come and go suddenly.
■ Jerking, twitching movements.

Mental/emotional

■ Anxious.
■ Delirious, raving, restless, excitable.
■ May lash out when hallucinating.
■ All senses heightened and easily aggravated.
■ Craves lemons.

Modalities

Worse: mid-afternoon and during the night. Throbbing headache worse for bending down; worse for anything which affects the senses; heat, touch, light, noise, smell, movement, sudden temperature changes.

Better: at rest; with minimal stimulation; for cold drinks once fever subsided.

Look for different remedy if . . .

Slow onset. Ongoing, chronic condition. Has fear of death. Calm.

Also consider . . .

Aconite; Bryonia; and other remedies according to notable symptoms.

Bryonia (Bryonia Alba)

Usual abbreviation: **Bryonia or Bry**

 Worse any movement

 Thirst, cold drinks

 Better holds affected part

 Dry, parched

Remedy made from the roots of the hedgerow plant, white bryony (wild hops) before it blooms. *Caution: The plant in its natural state is extremely poisonous.*

Key words

Irritability; chest infections; dryness; great thirst for cold drinks; acute headaches which affect eyes; headache accompanies other conditions; worse for movement.

Possible precipitating situations

Changeable weather conditions, especially from cold to warm. Often at the change of seasons. Becoming chilled after perspiring from effort. Money worries.

Main signs and symptoms

General/physical

- Slow onset over several days.
- Acute headaches, pain behind eyes.
- Dry mouth, lips and mucous membranes.
- Great thirst to alleviate dryness.
- Face appears deep red colour.
- Aggravated by movement.
- Digestive upsets; constipation.

Mental/emotional

- Irritable, angry, anxious, sullen.
- Confused, indecisive, stupefied.
- Normally of a controlling and methodical nature.
- Wants to be left alone.

Modalities

Better: for pressure; may hold, or bind the affected part to gain relief. For dry weather, if eyes are closed; if allowed to rest undisturbed; for cold; for lying on affected side.
Worse: for heat; lack of fresh air. Pains intensified by any movement.

Look for different remedy if . . .

Fearful, with morbid thoughts. Restless and better for movement. No thirst.

Also consider . . .

Aconite;Arsenicum Album; Belladonna; Gelsemium; Rhus Toxicodendron; and other remedies according to notable symptoms.

Calcarea Carbonica

Usual abbreviation: Calc-C

Better dry weather

 Chilly but sweaty

All waste sour/offensive

Craves candy, chalk, coal, eggs

Remedy made from part of the shell of the European edible oyster; or from carbonate of lime (limestone).

Key words

Soon exhausted. Stubborn, yet indecisive and shy. Large appetite, craves eggs and sweets, dislikes meat, milk, may be overweight. Easily catches colds. Chilly type. Congestions. Varicosed or haemorrhoidal veins.

Possible precipitating situations

Developmental delay in growth; walking or talking; in children. Adult symptoms arise after exposure to cold water, or cold, damp weather. Person who easily catches a cold.

Main signs and symptoms

General/physical

- Tendency to frequent colds.
- Cravings: eggs; chalk; coal; sweets.
- Congestions; sluggish metabolism; constipation; poor circulation.
- Feels chilly, perhaps with patchy sweating, especially of the head area.
- Perspires after minimal effort.
- Malaise and weakness.
- Swollen and sore glands which feel hard.
- Legs and feet especially cold.
- Sour-smelling breath, sweat, flatulence, vomiting and diarrhoea.
- Disabling headache from suppressed cold symptoms.
- Chronic sore throat making swallowing difficult.

Mental/emotional

- ■ Stubborn and difficult, easily tired by mental endeavour.
- ■ Fearful and despairing.
- ■ Wilful and disobedient child, clumsy and slow to learn.
- ■ Feigns indifference to mask inability to make decisions.
- ■ Feels trapped and hemmed in by own indecisiveness.
- ■ Sensitive to criticism.
- ■ Child easily takes fright or offence.
- ■ Slow to move; slumps when seated; pale appearance.
- ■ Sour-smelling cradle cap on infant's head.

Modalites

Worse: for exposure to damp or cold air; when baby is teething; after physical exertion; when standing; for mental effort; when watched; if menstruating; diarrhoea worse after mid-day.
Better: for warm, dry conditions; for lying down; when constipated.

Look for different remedy if . . .

Better for opening bowels, for movement, or for sunlight. Worse for warmth.

Also consider . . .

Chamomilla; Pulsatilla; Silica; and other remedies according to notable symptoms.

Calendula (Calendula officinalis)

Usual abbreviation: Cal

The remedy is made from the flowers and tips of the pot marigold plant.

Key words

Minor wounds, cuts or abrasions when skin is broken.

NB: Available in the form of cream, ointment, oil or tincture, Calendula is usually applied externally. In this respect it does not meet the strictest criteria for a homeopathic remedy as the external treatment of local symptoms can cause suppression of disease. However, as it may be obtained prepared to homeopathic principles, it is included in this list. It is one of the most useful items in the medicine cabinet for the external treatment of wounds and abrasions, promoting healing without scarring or infection. It is invaluable in emergency first-aid situations which involve broken skin, when Arnica cannot be applied.

Possible precipitating situations

Cuts, lacerations, abrasions, wounds. Following dental treatment as a dilute mouthwash; following childbirth – natural, caesarian section, episiotomy. Promotes healing without scars.

Main signs and symptoms

General/physical

- Open wounds, cuts and grazes.
- Cracked and abraded skin.
- Cracked nipples (remove cream before breastfeeding and reapply after).
- Following dental treatment (dilute mouthwash).
- Nappy/diaper rash.
- Later treatment of burns when needing to promote new tissue growth.

Mental/emotional

None.

Modalities

None.

Look for different remedy if . . .

Need to take remedy internally, such as Arnica for shock. Seeking immediate treatment for burns. In cases of major trauma, seek professional help.

Also consider . . .

Arnica, if the skin is not broken; Cantharis; Hamamelis; Rhus Toxicodendron; and other remedies according to notable symptoms.

Cantharis (Cantharis Vesicatoria)

Usual abbreviation: Canth

 Sudden onset

 Great thirst

Burning pains, inflammations

Worse for touch

Remedy made from the insect, Lytta Vesicatoria, otherwise known as Spanish fly, or blister beetle.

Key words

Burning pains, actual burns or scalds before blisters emerge, sunburn, burning sensation when urinating or in the bladder, insect bites. Worse for cold drinks despite thirst. Urinary inflammations.

Possible precipitating situations

Burns, sunburn; blisters; non-specific urinary infections; insect bites. NB: Seek help if condition worsens, as these symptoms may lead to serious complaints such as kidney failure and loss of consciousness, beyond the scope of amateur prescribing.

Main signs and symptoms

General/physical

- Rapid onset of burning pains, especially affecting urinary or sexual organs.
- Painful, burning cystitis, before, during and after urination.
- Pains anywhere of a burning, scalding nature.

- Burned or scalded skin; raging inflammations.
- Extreme restlessness.
- Frequent desire to urinate, but to little effect.
- Unable to swallow liquids.
- Dislike of bright light.
- Right-sided pain predominates.
- Blood in urine.

Mental/emotional

- Excitable, restless, confused.
- Anger, mania.

Modalities

Worse: for drinking, especially cold drinks or coffee, despite burning thirst; if touched.
Better: for warmth and rest; for cold applications.

Look for different remedy if . . .

Pain-free urination. Pain even when not urinating. Stress incontinence. Onset gradual. Precipitated by exposure to cold or a shock. Urinary pain accompanied by discharge. Improved by cold bathing or cold drinks.

Also consider . . .

Aconite; Apis Mellifica; Arsenicum Album; Lycopodium; Pulsatilla; Sepia; Staphysagria; and other remedies according to notable symptoms. NB: You may need to consult a larger Materia Medica to be sure of the correct remedy for the many specific cystitis symptoms.

Carbo Veg (Carbo Vegetabilis)

Usual abbreviation: Carb-V

 Chilly

Better for being fanned

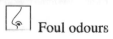 Foul odours

Worse for fatty foods

Remedy made from wood charcoal. Sometimes called the *corpse reviver*.

Key words

Dyspepsia and flatulence temporarily eased by belching. Collapse, including cases of carbon monoxide poisoning (having first summoned professional help). Violent coughing. Cold skin and cold sweats but needs fanning. Head warm. Exhaustion.

Possible precipitating situations

Shock or trauma. Pregnancy when baby is high in the womb. Aged, especially if infirm and weak. Overindulgence. Following incomplete recovery from the measles or whooping cough. May be used in extreme emergency until professional help arrives, following carbon monoxide poisoning from car exhaust, or malfunctioning gas appliances; for a newborn baby, if blue-tinged and cold from a protracted labour, or an elderly person found cold and collapsed. *NB: Always call the emergency services for help before starting to treat for collapse, or suspected carbon monoxide poisoning.*

Main signs and symptoms

General/physical

- Collapse or near collapse from extreme exhaustion.
- Extreme tiredness after respiratory illness, measles or whooping cough.
- Digestive disturbances; trapped wind, leading to belching.
- Bloated, distended stomach and malodorous breath and flatulence.
- Hiccoughs.
- Chesty cough will accompany a cold in Carb-V type.
- Poor circulation leading to weakness, blue extremities, and cold skin.
- Desires to be fanned although feels cold.
- Warm head.

Mental/emotional

- Cravings: for salt, sugary foods, stimulants such as tea, coffee, alcohol.
- Aversion to fatty foods and milk products.
- Lacking vitality and despondent, yet quickly rouses to anger and tears.
- Fears, especially of occult phenomena, and of the dark.
- Short-term memory impairment.
- Suicidal ideation is possible.

Modalities

Worse: for greasy/fatty foods, which cause flatulence; for warmth.
Better: for fresh air; for belching.

Look for different remedy if . . .

Weakness is associated with fearful anticipations, or follows from a loss of fluids.

Also consider . . .

Argentum Nitricum; Lycopodium. You may need to consult a larger Materia Medica to be sure of the correct remedy for specific symptoms other than those mentioned here.

Chamomilla (Matricaria Chamomilla)

Usual abbreviation: **Cham**

 Shrieks with temper/pain

 Craves cold drinks; worse stimulants

Worse for touch but better carried

Remedy made from the plant, wild chamomile, when in flower. Also known as German chamomile and corn feverfew. NB: Overuse of chamomile as a herbal tea may actually prove or cause these same symptoms.

Key words

Cries out with unbearable pain. Labour pains. Teething. Oversensitive to pain, temperamental, impatient, angry, inconsolable. Child prefers to be carried.

Possible precipitating situations

Teething infant, infant colic. Anger. After consuming coffee or an excess of chamomile tea. Psychological distress. Labour pains.

Main signs and symptoms

General/physical

- Unbearable pain causing tearful, griping distress.
- Shouts, cries, screams or moans from pain and frustration.
- Unable to sleep due to pain or coughing. Bad dreams.
- Lashes out in frustration and anger.
- Head hot and moist to the touch.
- Red faced.
- Thirst for cold drinks.
- Colicky pain perhaps with offensive flatulence, diarrhoea.
- Sensitive and tender, resists touch and being covered.
- Disproportionate over-reaction to pain.
- Earache very sensitive to cold air.
- Numb from pain.

Mental/emotional

- Irritable, angry, frenzied and impossible to pacify.
- Oversensitive, particularly to pain.
- Impatient, intolerant, easily offended.

Modalities

Worse: for attention, touch; if exposed to draughts, wind, damp; after drinking coffee; at night. Pains often worse for heat, but not made better by cold.

Better: infant better for being carried or transported, and for rocking movement. Colic better for local warmth, and for knees raised towards chest.

Look for different remedy if . . .

Infant arches back with colic pain – colic improved by doubling up, or for firm pressure. Nausea, diarrhoea and dyspepsia present; and according to specific symptoms presented.

Also consider . . .

Nux vomica; and other remedies, according to notable symptoms, some beyond the scope of this book. Chamomilla is not the sole remedy for the fractious child.

Cuprum Met. (Cuprum Metallicum)

Usual abbreviation: Cupr

 Metallic taste   Worse hot weather

 Excitable/changeable   Spasmodic cramps/seizures

Remedy made from the poisonous metallic element, copper, which is essential for health in the form of a trace element.

Key words

Extremely contrasting symptoms every half hour. Cramps. Spasms, seizures, twitches. Metallic taste. Pale face, blue lips. Extreme mood changes. *NB: Seek immediate professional medical help before treatment for any patient having convulsions or chest pains.*

Possible precipitating situations

Childhood teething; cramps following childbirth; menopause (when supported by wider symptom picture); tension (PMT) from delayed menstruation.

Main signs and symptoms

General/physical

- Symptoms appear grouped together, every half hour or so alternating through extreme contrasts.
- Spasmodic, cramping, jerking pains followed by exhaustion.
- Profound sleep during which violent spasms and twitches.
- Painful spasms, start at extremities which feel cold, and move upwards.
- Metallic taste.
- Violent stomach cramps.
- Convulsions, blue lips, cramping pains – **seek professional help**.
- Coughing fit induces spasms and twitching extremities alternating with loss of breath, then rapid panting – **seek professional help**.
- Headache from lack of sleep and mental exhaustion.
- Great hunger followed by aversion to food.
- Itchy spots pimples and ulcers.
- Excessive vomiting and nausea.
- Vertigo.
- Calf muscles knotted in cramping spasms.

Mental/emotional

- Highly strung, edgy and excitable.
- Moods contradictory and extremely changeable.

Modalities

Better: if can be encouraged to relax. Spasms better for pressure; cough better for drinking a little cold water. Better for sweating.
Worse: at evening and night; for exposure to cold air; for touch; for hot weather and sunlight; after vomiting; if discharges are suppressed, as in a delay or failure to menstruate.

Look for different remedy if . . .

Cramps persistent rather than spasmodic; stomach, leg or chest pains without cramping spasms; temperament even and unchanging.

Also consider . . .

Rhus toxicodendron; Mercurius; and other remedies beyond the scope of this book, according to notable symptoms.

Drosera (Drosera Rotundifolia)

Usual abbreviation: Dros

 Worse warmth   Better for fresh air

Worse after midnight

Remedy made from complete round-leaved sundew plant when ready to flower.

Key words

Tickly, spasmodic cough. Worse lying down.

Possible precipitating situations

Whooping cough; family history of tuberculosis.

Main signs and symptoms

General/physical

- Dry, painful cough; whooping cough.
- Throat tickles making swallowing difficult; voice hoarse and deep.
- Cough in spasms, causing retching and even vomiting.
- Nosebleed precipitated by coughing.
- Aching limbs.
- Face hot while extremities cold and shivering.

Mental/emotional

■ Restless, anxious, with poor concentration.
■ Quick to anger; easily slighted and suspicious.
■ Feels victimized and cheated.

Modalities

Worse: for lying down; after midnight; for drinking or talking; warmth; for movement; chest pain worse for coughing.
Better: for fresh air; if pressure applied; if holds chest when coughing.

Look for different remedy if . . .

Cough is accompanied with continuous nausea; in a state of exhausted collapse from coughing; if face is very red; if better for warmth, worse for fresh air; if hallucinating and craves lemons.

Also consider . . .

Belladonna; Carbo Vegetabilis; Ipecacuanha; and other remedies according to notable symptoms.

Eupatorium Perfoliata

Usual abbreviation: Eup-P

 Bones ache as if broken

Chill 7–9 am after bone-ache

Restless yet worse for movement

Remedy made from vegetable antimony (agueweed; boneset) when in flower.

Key words

Restless fever, cold, or influenza; aching bones, eyes and scalp. Sleepiness. Laboured breathing. Raised shoulders, hands on knees, to support the chest and assist breathing. Shivers, chills. Thirst for cold drinks. Sweat scanty.

Possible precipitating situations

Influenza; cold; fever.

Main signs and symptoms

General/physical

Feels sore, bones ache as if broken. Chill at 7–9 am after bones ached.

Very restless to escape pains though wishes to be still.

Feels chilly and desires warmth.

Great thirst for cold drinks.

Nausea and vomiting after the chill.

Dry, painful cough with a sore chest.

■ Back of head aches and throbs and is made worse by sweating.

Great desire to sleep.

Aching eyes and scalp, bones ache and feel as though broken, chills and shivers, sneezing, catarrh, bursting headache.

Fever symptoms may progress to biliousness and even jaundice.

Breathing difficult and laboured, characteristic position of raised shoulders with hands on knees to support the chest and assist breathing.

Mental/emotional

Depression and sadness accompanying winter cold.

Restless anxiety.

Modalities

Better: for sweating, except with headache which is made worse by it; for cold air.
Worse: for movement; if cold water drunk during the chill.

Look for different remedy if . . .

Patient remains still rather than restless with pain.

Illness precipitates anger rather than depression and sadness.

Also consider . . .

Bryonia; Nux Vomica; and other remedies according to notable symptoms.

Euphrasia (Euphrasia Officinalis)

Usual abbreviation: Euphr

Remedy made from the eyebright plant.

 Worse for sunlight   Worse for warmth

Eyes affected

Key words

Streaming cold, profuse discharges; stinging, watery eyes. Chills. Averse to bright light.

Possible precipitating situations

The group of symptoms usually associated with a head cold, hay fever, and eye complaints such as conjunctivitis and blepharitis.

Main signs and symptoms

General/physical

- Feels cold and cannot be warmed.
- Catarrhal headache.
- Copious burning, watery discharge from eyes makes skin sore, eyes sting.
- Inflamed, swollen, reddened and itchy eyes and lids.
- Bland nasal discharge; sneezing.
- Catarrh.
- Bursting headache affecting sight.

- Fever mainly during the day.
- Red face, cold hands.
- Loose, productive cough, generally; rarely a dry cough, but absent at night.

Mental/emotional

None of note.

Modalities

Better: if lying down; for bathing eyes.
Worse: for warmth and in the evening. Head cold symptoms worse at night. Cough worse for reclining and in the daytime. Eyes worse for bright light, for sunlight, wind or cold air.

Look for different remedy if . . .

Cough maintained through the night.

Also consider . . .

Allium Cepa; Arsenicum Album; Bryonia; Gelsemium; Mercurius Solubilis; Natrum Muriaticum; Pulsatilla; and other remedies according to notable symptoms.

Gelsemium (Gelsemium Sempervirens)

Usual abbreviation: Gels

 Slow onset

 Anticipatory anxiety

 Worse for heat of the sun

 Thirst absent

Remedy made from the bark of the rhizome and roots of the yellow (or false) Jasmine plant. *Caution: This plant is poisonous if consumed in excess.*

Key words

Influenza; trembling; congestive headache. Chills despite fever. Glassy eyes. Absence of thirst. Fearful and introverted.

Possible precipitating situations

Following bad news, shame, fear or embarrassment. After a shock or fright particularly if accompanied with trembling. An overheated environment. Climatic changes.

Main signs and symptoms

General/physical

- Gradual onset.
- Congestive complaints, especially constricting headaches, colds, influenza, constipation.
- Extreme exhaustion, sense of heaviness, and mental confusion.
- Face purple or red.
- Skin blotchy.
- Eyes glassy sometimes with dilated pupils, heavy lidded. Vision blurred.
- Cold extremities, chills with great fever.
- Diarrhoea following emotional state.
- Absence of thirst.
- Frequent urination.
- Sleepy.

Mental/emotional

- Depression without weeping.
- Fearful of crowds, examinations, tests or public speaking.
- Prefers to be alone.
- Fear of the dark.
- Sensory disturbances.

Modalities

Better: for lying down, moderate warmth; for pressure to area of congestion; for urinating and for sweating; after consuming alcohol.

Worse: for movement and over-heated environment.

Look for different remedy if . . .

Great thirst, sudden onset.

Also consider . . .

Aconite; Belladonna; Bryonia; and other remedies beyond the scope of this book according to notable symptoms.

Hamamelis (Hamamelis Virginica)

Usual abbreviation: Ham

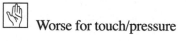 Worse for touch/pressure   Worse for drinking water

Worse for fresh air   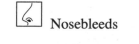 Nosebleeds

Remedy made from the bark of the Witch Hazel tree (spotted alder). NB: Available as cream and ointment for external application as well as standard homeopathic remedy for internal treatment.

Key words

Congested veins; haemorrhage after injury. Bruising.

Possible precipitating situations

Haemorrhage following injury or tooth extraction. Pregnancy or childbirth leading to varicose veins or haemorrhoids (piles). Family history of varicosed veins.

Main signs and symptoms

General/physical

- Sore and bruised.
- External bleeding, dark blood.
- Varicose veins, anywhere.
- Bruising around the eye (black eye) affecting sight.
- Persistent nosebleed or bleeding gums.

Mental/emotional

None of note.

Modalities

Worse: for touch of bruises or source of bleeding; nosebleeds worse in the morning, for drinking water, which causes nausea; for fresh air.
Better: still and quiet; lying down.

Look for different remedy if . . .

Thirsts for water. Better for touching affected area. Recurrent nosebleeds without precipitating injury. Nosebleed with whooping cough symptoms. Nosebleed following violent coughing fit which caused choking or vomiting. Nosebleed is not profuse but is bright red. Better for open air when has menstrual problems. Nose burns and itches when bleeding.

Also consider . . .

Arnica (if skin is broken take internally only); Carbo Vegetabilis; Drosera; Ipecacuanha; Phosphorus; Pulsatilla; Sulphur; and other remedies according to notable symptoms.

Hepar Sulph (Hepar Sulphuris Calcareum)

Usual abbreviation: Hep-S

 Worse any sensations   Better wet weather

 Better warmth   Feels chilly

Remedy made from the mineral calcium sulphide (obtained from powdered oyster shells and flowers of sulphur in equal measure).

Key words

Hypersensitive senses. Suppurating wounds. Unpleasant body odours. Throat sore, as if splintered. Wheezy. Lower lip cracked. Swollen glands. Chilly.

Possible precipitating situations

Exposure to a cold, dry wind.

Main signs and symptoms

General/physical

■ Abscesses (glandular and dental) pus-filled and painfully sensitive to touch (splintering pain).

Childhood croup, worse in early morning after exposure to cold.

■ Hypersensitive to heat, cold, pain, smell, touch, sound, air currents.

Rapid onset of symptoms which may affect ears, nose, throat, lungs.

■ Easily catches colds and feels chilly.

Severe, splintering pains.

■ Dry, tickly, productive cough and painful throat as if swallowed needles.

Glands swollen and inflamed.

Catarrh and hoarseness.

Profuse, smelly discharges; all bodily waste smells sour and cheesy.

■ Sweats at night.

Symptoms worsen very quickly if any part of the body uncovered.

Suppurating skin infections (boils, spots, pimples) which are slow to heal.

■ Headache right-sided; pains at the base of nose on the right side.

■ Angered by being touched and will block attempts to elicit information.

Speaks and eats rapidly.

Mental/emotional

- Hypersensitive, irritable, demanding, abusive and quickly angered.
- Impetuous and impulsive.
- Finds fault with everything and everyone.
- Easily bored, craves constant change.
- Cravings for acidic food and drink, with aversion for fatty foods.

Modalities

Better: for warmth and warm drinks; for wet weather.
Worse: for touch, draughts, and cold; if lies on affected side; for tight, restrictive clothing. Headache made worse by movement.

Look for different remedy if . . .

The discharges are thin and caustic and do not smell offensive; even temperament; overwhelming fears and anxieties; croup worse in the evening.

Also consider . . .

Aconite; Argentum Nitricum; Mercurius Solubilis; Silica; and other remedies according to notable symptoms.

Hypericum (Hypericum Perforatum)
Usual abbreviation: Hyp

 Worse for movement   Worse for touch

 Worse for cold air   Craves drinks/hot milk

Remedy made from the complete flowering plant, St. John's Wort.

Key words

Wounds, injuries or surgical interventions affecting neural pathways; puncture wounds; open wounds; blows to the head. Great pain, worse for movement. Nervous system.

Possible precipitating situations

Any injuries or wounds affecting the nerves, or nerve-rich areas; cuts, wounds, crushed fingers or toes, puncture wounds. Trauma especially if affecting the coccyx or lower back. Sciatica, neuralgia, shingles. Lumbar puncture. Childbirth: forceps or caesarian delivery; episiotomy. Animal or insect bites which cause shooting pains. Splinter(s) in skin. After any surgery when nerves inflamed and sore. NB: In a first-aid situation, reduce swelling with arnica before using hypericum, and also consider ledum for puncture wounds.

Main signs and symptoms

General/physical

- Severe, tearing, shooting pains along nerve path.
- Bruising and soreness; laceration; puncture; open wounds.
- Crushed or torn nail bed.
- Injury to the head: concussion.
- Pain in coccyx or lower back ascends the spine.
- Bites (animal or insect) which affect the nerves.
- Splintered skin which is painful and inflamed.
- Painful old scars.
- Wants to drink hot milk.

Mental/emotional

- Shock arising from injuries to the nerves.
- Memory loss and drepression.

Modalities

Worse: if pressure applied; for cold environment, cold air, and for touch or movement.

Better: if rests on affected side.

Look for different remedy if . . .

Pain slight and wounds superficial. Nerves not affected. Need to prevent bruising or swelling use arnica before giving hypericum, where indicated.

Also consider . . .

Arnica to reduce swelling (taken internally where skin is broken); Calendula; Ledum Palustre (for initial treatment of bites); and other remedies according to notable symptoms.

Ignatia (Ignatia Amara)

Usual abbreviation: Ign

 Worse for inhaling smoke   Better eating

Worse for sweets/candy    After emotional upheaval/sighs

Remedy made from the seeds of the St. Ignatius bean plant. *Caution: The St. Ignatius bean is poisonous unless homeopathically prepared.*

Key words

Strong emotional upset. Suppressed emotions. Eating disorders. Insomnia.

Possible precipitating situations

A sense of loss or worry. Death, accident, critical illness or loss of a loved one. Shock of rejection, punishment or censure. Emotionally slighted. Examination nerves. Intense jealousy. Acute disappointment. Heartbroken. Homesickness. The suppression of strong emotions.

Main signs and symptoms

General/physical

Variable emotional and physical states; all symptoms changeable.

Silent; brooding; tearful; anguished; enraged; hysterical; inconsolable grief.

Large sighs; frequent yawning.

■ Spasms, twitching and shaking.

Tension headaches; feeling that head is being pierced.

Deafness; roaring sounds or sensation of having water in the ears.

■ Feels as if a lump in the throat; eased by eating.

Coughing fit leaves patient gasping.

■ Will not be comforted by touch or word. Prefers to be alone.

Acute illnesses which follow soon after shock or grief.

Emotionally triggered eating disorders such as anorexia nervosa/bulimia.

Appetite disturbed; disinterest in food; overeating.

■ Craving for raw, indigestible foods. Aversion to milk and fruit.

Thirst when feels cold but none when feels hot.

Mental/emotional

Mood swings: sobbing; silent tears; withdrawn and sad.

Irritable, impatient and intolerant, angry.

Nightmares; insomnia; sleepwalking.

Desire to be alone.

Sensitive type who tends to hide emotions rather than express them.

Modalities

Worse: for touch and for fresh air; for coffee, for sweets and candies; for inhaling tobacco smoke.
Better: if takes deep breaths; for eating or drinking; for heat.

Look for different remedy if . . .

The symptoms resulting from emotional shock are physical, not emotional; the cause of emotional upset is not recent; unexpressed humiliation predominates; there is no emotion; primarily anticipatory anxiety; craves company.

Also consider . . .

Argentum Nitricum; Natrum Muriaticum; Pulsatilla; Sepia; Staphysagria; consult a larger Materia Medica for other remedies according to symptoms. NB: Seek professional counselling and medical help for serious eating disorders.

Ipecac (Ipecacuanha)

Usual abbreviation: Ip

 Thirst absent   Worse for food

Temperamental   Worse for warmth

Remedy made from the dried roots of the Brazilian Cephaelis Ipecacuanha plant, collected when in flower.

Key words

Nausea and vomiting in addition to other complaint(s). Rapid onset, cyclic symptoms; choking; breathing difficulties.

Possible precipitating situations

Following: anger or frustration, suppressed emotion; diarrhoea or nausea from over eating; childbirth. Any complaint when it is accompanied with nausea and vomiting.

Main signs and symptoms

General/physical

■ Onset within a few hours.

■ Symptoms occur in a regular periodic cycle alternating with prostration.

■ Nausea and vomiting with another complaint(s), particularly coughs or bronchitis.

■ Difficulty breathing causing face to become blue-tinged, reddened or pale.

■ Breathing rapid with wheezing.

■ Persistent, dry coughing fits causing gasps for air and sudden vomiting.

■ Child who stiffens and turns blue from violent coughing.

■ Hot or cold sweats; violent chills.

■ Cold with stuffed up nose; inability to cough up mucus from chest.

■ Constipation.

■ Diarrhoea, stools or vomit green in colour.

■ Blood in mucus and sputum.

Mental/emotional

■ Demanding, irritable, angry, highly critical and scornful of others.

■ Child has tantrum to get what it wants, but impossible to please.

Modalities

Better: for fresh air and from sitting erect; for cold drinks.
Worse: for cold, humidity or warmth; for rich or fatty foods; for the smell of food or tobacco smoke; at night.

Look for different remedy if . . .

Nausea is relieved by vomiting. Continuous prostration. Great thirst without accompanying fever.

Also consider . . .

Arsenicum; Kalium Bichromium; Pulsatilla; Sepia; and other remedies according to notable symptoms.

Kali Bich (Kalium Bichromicum)

Usual abbreviation: Kali-B

 Worse 2–3 am

 Slow onset

Better for movement

 Worse for cold weather

Remedy made from the mineral Potassium Chromate (Bichromate of potash) extracted from chromium iron ore.

Key words

Symptoms follow change in the weather. Sinus conditions. Catarrh. Migraine.

Possible precipitating situations

Chilly person who takes colds and chills easily; after exposure to cold or changeable weather. Person whose colds tend to affect the sinuses.

Main signs and symptoms

General/physical

■ Chronic catarrh.

■ Nasal discharge thick, dry, crusty, leaves sores if removed, then re-crusts.

■ Plentiful yellow mucus discharge, thick, stringy or jellified, from any mucous membranes in the body (nose, throat, chest, stomach and intestines, vagina, urethra.).

■ Pains come and go in different places, changing rapidly.

Acute pain concentrated in small areas of a few centimetres.

■ Ulcerated mucous membranes, especially of the throat.

Slow onset of symptoms.

Tongue has yellow or white coating.

Catarrh symptom alternates with diarrhoea or rheumatic joint pains.

Nasal discharge dries in cold air to be replaced with throbbing headache.

Headache localized in small spots, sight affected, occurs at regular times.

Earache, worse on left side, with thick, yellow discharge.

Throat severely inflamed with swollen tonsils.

Wheezy, dry cough causing pain from chest through to back.

Pain at base of the spine and between shoulder blades.

Mental/emotional

Lacks vitality, feels tired, weak and listless.

Distrustful of others.

Mental (and physical) performance impaired, no desire to make effort.

Modalities

Better: for warmth and rest; pressure on headache or sinus pain. Usually better for movement but headache worse for bending/ movement.

Worse: in the early morning, 2–3 am; for cold or changeable weather. Cough worse for breathing and damp, or cold weather.

Look for different remedy if . . .

Discharges are excoriating and are green rather than yellow. Affected by heat or by cold, preferring median temperatures. Tearful, needs emotional support; clingy. Better for cold air.

Also consider . . .

Belladonna; Mercurius Solubilis; Pulsatilla; and other remedies according to notable symptoms.

Ledum Palustre (Ledum)

Usual abbreviation: Led

 Worse warmth even if feels cold

 Better cold/cold applications

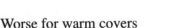 Worse for warm covers

Worse at night

Remedy made from the whole Marsh Tea Herb (wild rosemary shrub).

Key words

Puncture wounds; animal bites, mosquito bites and stings, wandering pains; black eye. *NB: If punctured by soiled implements or an animal bite seek urgent professional help for the risk of tetanus or rabies infections.*

Possible precipitating situations

Puncture wounds, nails, thorns, etc. Bites and stings. Injured, painful joints. A blow to the eye region causing a black eye. May be used as a preventative for those who habitually react stongly to bites and stings.

Main signs and symptoms

General/physical

- Swollen, painful joints; sprained ankle, wrist; injured tendons affecting mobility when legs or feet affected.
- Bites, stings, puncture wounds painful to the touch, infected, swollen.
- Individual feels cold, chilly.

■ Blackened or bruised and swollen eye; bloodshot, following injury.

■ Thirsty for cold water.

Mental/emotional

■ Self pitying.

■ Disturbed dreams.

Modalities

Better: for cold compress, cold bathing, even if complains of feeling cold.

Worse: for warm room, warm covers, even though feels cool; for movement of puncture site or injured joint; at night; for drinking alcohol, though craves it.

Look for different remedy if . . .

Bites and stings swollen; hot; red and shiny, very itchy. Joints swollen, hot and red. Injuries where skin is not broken, and need for help is rejected or denied. Simple cuts and abrasions. Injury to nerve tissue. Pain on site of injection. Sharp, needling pains. Pains better for application of heat, worse for cold. Restless, better for movement.

Also consider . . .

Apis Mellifica; Arnica; Calendula; Hypericum; Rhus Toxicodendron; Ruta Graveolens; and other remedies according to notable symptoms.

Lycopodium (Lycopodium Clavatum)

Usual abbreviation: Lyc

R-side pain, may cross to L

Worse 4–8 pm, or at set times

 Loss of appetite

 Dryness

Remedy made from the fruiting spores of Club Moss, also called Stag's Horn and Wolf's Claw.

Key words

Emotional fears. Deep lines in forehead and face which is pale. Prematurely aged. Weakness. Sour sweats. Digestive symptoms, with excess gas. Worse at set times. Sweet tooth. Chilly.

Possible precipitating situations

Imminent change to routine or challenge to competence. On waking.

Main signs and symptoms

General/physical

- Chronc tiredness.
- Symptoms worsen at predictable times, e.g. between 4 and 8 pm.
- Bloated with gas. Poor digestion, soon replete, or loss of appetite.
- Dry, congested sinuses and nasal crustiness with common cold. Ears congested.
- Catarrhal eye conditions.
- Mouth breathing when nasally congested.
- Slow onset.
- Right-sided pains; may cross to the left later; or from above to below.
- Sore throat or swollen glands which begin right-sided.
- Dry tickly cough; salty, yellow discharges and mucus.
- Throbbing headache, especially if food delayed.
- Craves sweets and chocolates.
- Symptoms mostly mental rather than physical.
- Insomnia due to anxieties.
- Constipation, or hard stools. Flatulence.

Mental/emotional

- Intellectual; likes to be right.
- Shy, hides lack of confidence with pretence of confidence.
- Self-doubt, feelings of inadequacy and low self-esteem.

- Fears being alone, fears humiliation.
- Fears change, fears exposure to risk or judgement, needlessly.
- Moody and difficult.
- Forgetful, indecisive.
- Depressed and irritable on waking.
- Depressed or angry if contradicted.
- Mental restlessness, poor concentration.

Modalities

Worse: on waking; at set time, e.g. 4–8 pm; for cold drinks or foods; for eating shellfish or brassicas; for eating legumes, breads, pastries and milk; for eating before an event; for pressure or tight clothing; airless room.

Better: for warmth, except head symptoms which are better for cold; hot drinks; for movement; for belching and flatulence; for urinating; for fresh air; loose clothing.

Look for different remedy if . . .

Impetuous; oversensitive; feels cold and thirsty; no digestive symptoms; unaffected by eating shellfish; calmly confident.

Also consider . . .

Argentum Nitricum; Natrum Muriaticum; Silica; and other remedies according to notable symptoms.

Merc (Mercurius)

Usual abbreviation: Merc

 Worse for cold weather   Worse for hot weather

 Thirst for cold drinks   Head hot/feels clamped

Remedy made from Mercury Oxide mixed with Nitric Acid, from the ore Cinnabar. There are many variations around the basic Merc remedy, each with slightly different properties. Mercury is naturally extremely toxic. It is often called quicksilver.

Key words

Unpleasant odours/breath/discharges/waste. Ulcers; abscesses. Metallic taste.

Possible precipitating situations

Recently exposed to change in temperature. Change of diet, water, environment.

Main signs and symptoms

General/physical

- Obvious and unpleasant smell emanates from all secretions/excretions.
- Glands become swollen, and irritated; membranes may be ulcerated.
- Profuse discharges; thin and burning, or thick, greeny/yellow, causing sores. Catarrh.
- Offensive breath; aching, bleeding gums; a metallic taste; tongue furred.
- Throat sore and appears swollen; difficulty swallowing.
- Foul-smelling urine and stools, possibly green-coloured diarrhoea.
- Suppurating sores, abscesses and infections which do not heal.
- Minor effort leads to a disproportionate exhaustion.
- Plentiful sweating though not hot. Feels chilled.
- Thirsts for cold drinks.
- Aversion for rich or spicy foods, sweets and candies, salt.
- Head feels hot and as though clamped in a band.
- Sensitive to light and fresh air.

Mental/emotional

- Withdrawn and non-communicative, unhappy. Confused and depressed.

■ Mercurial moods, though worse for change of any kind, including care.

■ A capricious, restless nature which does not take well to illness.

Modalities

Worse: at night and if lies on right side; for extremes of temperature; for change.
Better: in the morning and if lies on stomach.

Look for different remedy if . . .

Better for heat. Restless and feels better for change. Swollen glands with splinter-like pains. Extremely acute sensitivity to change. Emotionally accessible.

Also consider . . .

Arsenicum Album; Hepar Sulphuris Calcareum; and other remedies according to notable symptoms.

Nat Mur (Natrum Muriaticum)

Usual abbreviation: Nat-M

 Worse for sun/sunshine Dryness

 Worse mornings Great thirst

Remedy made from common rock salt (sodium chloride).

Key words

Typical sneezy cold. Herpes. Thirsts yet craves salt. Shy when urinating, at any age.

Possible precipitating situations

Sunstroke. Person habitually self-possessed and unlikely to express emotions, withdrawn, likely to suppress true feelings. After a reprimand or rejection. Grief. Prefers to suffer in silence. Imminent menstruation (with PMT).

Main signs and symptoms

General/physical

- Easily catches colds; start with lots of sneezing and runny nose; then dry.
- Dryness: cracked lips, dry skin, absence of saliva; bitter taste, great thirst.
- White-coloured discharges, whether thin and watery, or thick.
- Cannot urinate if accompanied/observed/in public, regardless of age.
- Resists weeping unless alone.
- Stitching, shooting pains.
- Lower back pain follows effort. Easily tired in general.
- Head hot and aching, nausea and vomiting, face red, after too much sun.
- Cold stores (herpes simplex) around the mouth after exposure to the sun.
- Blisters on the tongue.
- Children who are late in developing speech.
- Stools like small, dry pellets or copious, watery diarrhoea.
- Tickling, persistent cough which makes the eyes water.
- Head throbs when chilled, better for pressure, headache affects eyes*.
- Indigestion; hiccups/belching. Poor digestion; distended, gaseous bowel.
- Desires salty food despite great thirst.

*NB: If headaches are accompanied by visual disturbances seek urgent professional help.

Mental/emotional

- Inappropriate and misplaced emotional responses.
- Secretly stores up guilt feelings and instances of hurt. Brooding.
- Outwardly controlled, inwardly upset. Very unsettled by ridicule.
- Vague and confused, depressed and angry. Inconsolable.
- Vivid and disturbing dreams.

Modalities

Better: for est, sleep, and solitude; for fresh air but worse for draughts.
Worse: if overheated, better for sweating; in late morning; for exercise; for sympathy when upset.

Look for different remedy if . . .

Considerably worse for movement. Much sighing and emotional outpouring. High temperature and sudden onset of symptoms. No thirst. Even tempered.

Also consider . . .

Belladonna; Bryonia; Ignatia; and other remedies according to notable symptoms.

Nux Vom (Nux Vomica)

Usual abbreviation: Nux-V

 Craves stimulants/worse for them

 Worse 4 am

Worse for food

 Chilly/better for warmth

Remedy made from dried seeds of Strychnos Nux Vomica tree (Poison Nut or Quaker Buttons)

Key words

Excess: disturbed eating/sleeping pattern, over-indulgence, overwork. Fussy, irritable. Over-sensitive. Digestive upsets. No thirst. Imagines is ill.

Possible precipitating situations

Excess of: food, alcohol, stimulants, painkillers, work, mental or emotional stimulation. The classic hangover. After exposure to chill winds. Workaholic. Sleep disturbed by new baby.

Main signs and symptoms

General/physical

- Digestive upsets: bloat, heartburn, dyspepsia, constipation, diarrhoea.
- Nauseous but unable to vomit, or difficulty in vomiting. Retches.
- Hyper-sensitive: to pain, cold, light, smells and sounds.
- Headache centred over eyes, thumping pain on top of head. Dizzy.
- Inner ears itch beyond reach, relieved by swallowing.
- Frequent but incomplete evacuation of faeces. Frequent urge to urinate.
- Colds with frenzied sneezing, blocked sinuses, worse at night. hot sweats.
- Chills during fever.
- Needle-prick sore throat makes swallowing difficult.
- Dry, tickly, difficult cough; tight, painful chest; catches colds easily.
- Absence of thirst and chills when feverish.
- Back pains brought on by exposure to draught.
- Disturbed sleep, early morning insomnia.

Mental/emotional

- Easily angered, short tempered, hard to please; takes criticism badly.

■ Harried, but reluctant to delegate.

■ Aggressive rages; loss of control; imagined slights; spiteful.

■ Craves stimulants and spicy foods but upset by them.

■ Hyperchondriacal imaginings; over fastidious and tidy.

Modalities

Worse: for stimulants, for eating, for lack of sleep; at 4 am; on waking; after effort or mental exertion; for anger; for cold.
Better: for rest and sleep; warmth and cover; in evening; in damp weather; for defecating.

Look for different remedy if . . .

Fearful. Great thirst. Finds pains completely unbearable (more so than Rhus Tox). Distended with gas, eased with flatulence. Worse for warmth. Unaffected by spicy, rich food.

Also consider . . .

Arsenicum Album; Chamomilla; Lycopodium; Sulphur; and other remedies according to notable symptoms.

Phosphorus (Phosphorus)

Usual abbreviation: Phos

 Worse for cold weather   Better for eating

Fearful   Worse for bright light

Remedy made from the mineral, white phosphorus.

Key words

Low energy. Hot flushes. Bronchitis; lost voice; vomits especially after cold food/drink; bleeds easily. Palpitations.

Possible precipitating situations

Haemorrhaging after dental treatment. Menorrhagic. Acute hair loss if anaemic. Electrical storms. Youthful exhaustion after a period of rapid growth. Often fair-skinned, red-haired, tall and slim.

Main signs and symptoms

General/physical

- May affect any part of the body and its organization.
- Inflammations, especially of the blood, digestive and respiratory systems.
- Desperate need to eat.
- Great thirst for cold drinks. Warm drinks vomited.
- Searing, burning pains anywhere, especially the glands.
- Pains in digestive tract, may be relieved by eating cold food.
- Bleeds bright red blood profusely; slow to coagulate.
- Bleeds easily, blood may be present in sputum or other discharges.
- Dull, throbbing headache; headache localized over one eye.
- Tight chest, made worse by coughing; loss of voice and painful throat.
- The phosphorus cold typically alternates between exhibiting a runny nose and dry crusty nasal passages; one nostril is blocked and swollen while thin, bloody streaked mucus runs freely from the other.
- Hacking cough which is worse for fresh air.
- Feels cold, yet desires a cold environment and cool liquids to drink.
- Face and tongue may be flushed red and blotchy.
- Sensations of heat rising up the back or chest.
- Stools or diarrhoea may be blood streaked, but pain-free.

Mental/emotional

- Very sensitive, affectionate and empathetic. Craves company.
- Fearful, especially of death, of being left in the dark, or alone in a storm.
- Need for emotional contact may be great, or may be apathetic and cold.
- Slow, irritable, and mentally dulled when sick, unlike usual mental state.
- Desire to please, exhausts, then anger and irritation followed by remorse.

Modalities

Worse: for sensations: touch, bright light, smell; when emotionally aroused; when lies on the left side; and in the evenings; for changes in the weather or room temperature.

Better: for eating or drinking, especially if the food or drink is cold; for splashing cold water on face; for warm weather; for sleep, for massage of pain sites; for signs of affection.

Look for different remedy if . . .

Made worse by movement or touch. More thirsty than hungry. No thirst but emotionally clinging and weepy.

Also consider . . .

Bryonia; Pulsatilla; and other remedies according to notable symptoms.

Pulsatilla (Pulsatilla Nigricans)

Usual abbreviation: Puls

 Thirst absent though warm

 Better for fresh air

 Aversion to rich food

Face red

Remedy made from the flowering Pulsatilla Nigricans, the Windflower (also called Pasque Flower or Meadow Anemone).

Key words

No thirst. Tongue furred yellow/white, breath and sweat smells; worse for heat. Timid, anxious. Catarrhal complaints.

Possible precipitating situations

Cough. Cold, catarrh, earache, eye infection or teething child if pulsatilla-like in nature. Indigestion or stomach upset after rich or fatty foods. After getting wet, especially the feet. After measles. Emotional upsets; especially in adolescence. NB: Pulsatilla is effective for so many conditions (exceeded only by sulphur) that it has been given the nickname, the *Queen of Remedies*. Sulphur is nicknamed the *King of Remedies*. Any identifiable condition, or group of symptoms, may have pulsatilla characteristics which identify this remedy.

Main signs and symptoms

General/physical

- Mental and physical symptoms vary constantly, but always worse for heat.
- Symptoms disappear in fresh air, to reappear when deprived of it.
- Fever without thirst; all forms of warmth are rejected, even though chily.
- Dislike of wet and windy weather, and of being made wet accidentally.
- All discharges will be thick and yellow/green in appearance, but bland.
- Changeable desire for non-fatty, bland foodstuffs; yet craves butter.
- Characteristically, thirst will be absent.
- Mouth and lips dry; tongue furred; face flushed red.
- Awakes with bad taste in the mouth.

■ Insomnia from active mind. Rejects bed covers, yet awakens feeling cold.

■ Breath, flatulence and sweat smelly. May sweat in localized areas.

■ Headache throbs; often before menstruation. Cold compress improves.

■ Digestive upsets whenever ill, exacerbates by eating what will cause upset.

■ Lower back pains and sprains; joint pains which are better for compresses.

■ Frequent nosebleeds; atypical bed wetting.

■ Symptoms often one-sided.

Mental/emotional

■ A typically gentle and obliging person who craves attention when well.

■ Clingy and tearful when ill; needs comforting, more so in the evening.

■ Craves and gives affection; anticipates what will please to gain affection.

■ Restless, anxious, whiny and fussy, but not dramatic or hypersensitive.

■ Imagines is being excluded; jealous; becomes irritated; self-pitying, shy.

■ Empathy and fondness for animals and awareness of their needs.

Modalities

Worse: for heat, for warm clothing, environment, fatty food; for rest; for suppressed emotions. Digestive upsets worse in the morning.
Better: for fresh air and cold food and drink; for cool bath; gentle movement; for consoling and affection; for weeping.

Look for different remedy if . . .

Violent tantrums. Better for warmth, or worse for cold. Symptoms follow experience of mental upset. Mood swings and much sighing. Thick and stringy excoriating discharges. Great thirst.

Also consider . . .

Arsenicum Album; Ignatia; Kalium Bichromium; Phosphorus; and other remedies according to notable symptoms.

Rhus Tox (Rhus Toxicodendron)

Usual abbreviation: Rhus-T

 Better for movement after worse first

 Worse for cold/damp weather

Restlessness; physical/emotional

Worse for rest

Remedy made from leaves of the poison ivy plant before it flowers (also known as poison ash, poison oak, trailing sumach). The leaves are picked at night when the poison is most toxic. NB: Rhus Toxicodendron in its natural state can produce allergic skin reactions when touched by some individuals.

Key words

Restlessness; tongue red-tipped and sore; stiffness; joint pains and swellings; aggravated by cold; initially worse for gentle movement, then better for it, then tires and worsens as restlessness returns with inaction; acute thirst. Symptoms after exposure to cold/wet which chills or over-exertion.

Possible precipitating situations

Following surgical intervention, or injury. Swollen glands as with mumps; red, itchy rash as with chicken-pox if other symptoms match. After exposure to cold, draughts or wet conditions; from getting wet feet; changeable weather or following over-exertion, especially if sweating leads to a chill.

Main signs and symptoms

General/physical

■ Symptoms commonly begin at night.

Pain in joints and connective tissues and/or rash after becoming cold/wet.

Rheumaticky, aching pains in the back and neck.

Persistent fever, accompanied with chills. Hot then cold. Red faced.

Fever one-sided; alternate sides hot and cold.

Aches and sharp pains; weakened limbs which feel bruised or numb.

Sever cold symptoms with excoriating discharges which make skin sore.

Larynx and throat glands become swollen and sore. Ticklish cough.

Itchy, red heat rash just beneath the skin, sometimes itchy blisters.

Stultifying headache, as if clamped; eased by movement though neck stiff.

Ringing in the ears. Dizziness, sometimes affecting balance.

Restlessness; movement relieves, but soon exhausts, leading to necessary pause and renewed restlessness. Difficulty getting up.

Great thirst, but difficulty swallowing. Metallic taste.

Tongue furred yellowy white while tip is reddened and sore.

Cold food or drink seems to be felt instantly in the blood when feverish.

Frequent sweats over body (not the head) whether active or idle.

Mental/emotional

Mental restlessness, mild delirium, and anxiety when feverish.

Agitated dreams, irritability and night terrors; unhappy recollections at night.

Fearful of the motives of others; mild paranoia.

Tearful depression without clear cause.

■ Fears air travel for its restriction of movement and access to fresh air.

■ Desire to drink milk.

Modalities

Worse: for cold of any kind, even by touching a cold object or cold air; for cold drinks, or washing/swimming in cold water; headache worse by washing hair, or any wetting of the head. Worse for inadequate clothing or bed covers, for damp or draughts. Restlessness worse at night, eased by a walk in fresh air if warmly dressed; rash worse for scratching.

Better: for any heat; for hot baths; for rubbing the affected part; for sweating so long as not chilled by it; for warm drinks; for lying on a firm surface.

Look for different remedy if . . .

Strain brought on by overexertion is not relieved by continued gentle movement. Pains worse for any movement. Worse for warmth.

Also consider . . .

Apis Mellifica; Arnica; Belladonna; Bryonia; Ruta Graveolens; and other remedies according to notable symptoms.

Ruta Grav (Ruta Graveolens)

Usual abbreviation: Ruta

 Worse for cold weather

 Worse for windy weather

 Thirst for cold drinks

 Worse if moves affected parts

Remedy made from the common rue plant (bitter herb) before it flowers. NB: The herb Rue or Ruta Graveolens should be handled with caution in its natural state. It may cause allergic skin reactions.

Key words

Bone injuries. Sprained wrists or ankles. Pains of bruised character. Eye strain. Weakness.

Possible precipitating situations

Fractures of bones; strain injuries of joints, tendons and ligaments. Bruising. Musculoskeletal injuries which have failed to heal following acute treatment.

Main signs and symptoms

General/physical

    Site of injury (or exertion) aches, is tender and inflamed. Local swelling.

    Painful bones, especially the shins; joint pains.

    Joints remain weak after initial injury healed. Exercise aggravates.

    Eyes red and strained; aching and weak from overuse.

    Fibrous swellings at site of overexertion or repetitive strain.

    Fibrous swelling remains when bruising has healed.

■ Head aches as though were bruised and beaten.

    Cannot bear the weight of bedcovers pressing on affected part.

    Weak and weary.

    Great thirst for cold water.

Mental/emotional

    Restless, irritable and distrustful.

    Morbid fears.

    Self-critical and easily dissatisfied.

    Tearful, weary and depressed.

Modalities

Worse: for exertion; for pressure to, or for lying on the affected part; for draughts and wind; if exposed to cold or damp weather.

Better: for warmth and gentle movement; for lying on the back.

Look for different remedy if . . .

Pains over whole body, as if bruised. Worse for movement of any kind. Improved by exercise, after initial stiffness.

Also consider . . .

Arnica; Bryonia; Rhus Toxicodendron; and other remedies according to notable symptoms.

Sepia (Sepia)

Usual abbreviation: Sep

 Yellow bridge of nose/face

 Better for movement

Depressed/ uncommunicative

Craves sour foods

Remedy made from the ink of squid or cuttlefish.

Key words

Probably female; yellow face, discharges; hormonal disturbances; chilly; cold hands and feet; sweats easily; exhausted but better for energetic exercise; downcast; slack muscle tone; left-sided symptoms. *NB: Sepia strongly influences female hormones therefore although it can be beneficial for problems during pregnancy, or for a prolapsed uterus, in either case professional homeopathic advice must be sought.*

Possible precipitating situations

Largely applicable to women rather than men; menopausal and menstrual problems; postnatal problems; mother overtired by demands of children.

Main signs and symptoms

General/physical

Yellow face, especially bridge of the nose, dark circles beneath eyes.

Emotional upheavals; prone to weeping, irritability and depression.

■ Sweats easily; sour odours; sweats in particular area; cold or hot sweats.

Dispirited, apathetic, depressed and droops physically.

Hypersensitive to pain, to extreme heat or cold, and to loud music.

Left-sided symptoms predominate.

Dragging, dull. Aching pains.

Downward pressure on pelvis; tender, as if bruised.

Feels faint.

Yellow-white mucus which tastes salty.

Constipation, biliousness or thrush during pregnancy (consult homeopath).

Bedcoverings and warm clothes cause uneasiness.

Mental/emotional

Craving for sweets, vinegar, pickles and other sour foods.

Detached and unemotional when well.

Angry, anxious, irritable, depressed, sluggish, tearful when imbalanced.

Oblivious to needs of others when ill, usually cares for others when well.

Low libido.

■ Prefers to be alone; rejects help and sympathy.

Dislikes meat.

Modalities

Worse: for rest; for touch or massage; for lack of food; at night; for loud noises; for becoming cold or wet; before menstruation; for standing; for others' demands.

Better: for exercise despite lethargy; for eating; for being alone; for silence; for sitting up; for sleep; for keeping busy; for warmth, fresh air and sunshine.

Look for different remedy if . . .

Worse for exercise; fearful; craves salt; copious red blood and worse for heat; good skin tone and hue; communicative and desires company.

Also consider . . .

Natrum Muriaticum; Phosphorus; and other remedies beyond the scope of this materia medica, according to notable symptoms. *I suggest you always seek professional homeopathic advice before taking remedies when pregnant.*

Silica (Silicea)

Usual abbreviation: Sil

 After getting wet feet

 Slow to heal

Headache worse
bright light

 Worse for winter

Remedy made from Silicon Dioxide extracted from flint, quartz, rock crystal and sandstone.

Key words

Need for expulsion of physical matter; of foreign bodies; splinters, glass, thorns; abscesses, ulcers and boils; negative reactions to vaccinations. Icy cold. Thick, yellow discharges; catarrh.

Possible precipitating situations

Cold, damp weather, after getting wet feet. Vaccination(s).

Main signs and symptoms

General/physical

Taken internally to expel splinters, and other foreign bodies, even from eyes.

■ Infected wounds or broken bones which heal slowly.

Dental abscesses.

Suppressed discharges/sweat.

■ Ulcerated nipples; mastitis.

Swollen glands and lymph nodes.

■ Coldness which is resistant to warming.

Profuse, offensive sweat, especially at night of head, hands and feet.

Inner ear infections or perforated eardrums, better for yawning.

Offensive, thick and bloody discharge from ears.

Headaches start from back of head and move towards forehead/one eye.

Fontanelle slow to close in infancy. Slow teething.

Thirst.

Baby rejects mother's milk. Adult gets diarrhoea from drinking milk.

Faecal retention and difficulty in passing stools; stools retracted.

Flatulence.

Mental/emotional

Outwardly unassertive and sensitive in character yet inner resilience.

Fussy about personal appearance.

■ Mentally exhausted from overexertion. Poor concentration. Jumpy.

■ Prefers to duck responsibility and avoid effort, yet a very good worker.

■ Dislikes meat.

Modalities

Worse: for cold; for irregular meals; headache worse for sudden or loud noise, bright light; for being uncovered; for winter; for being comforted.
Better: for warmth, especially to the head; for cold food and drinks; for urinating.

Look for different remedy if . . .

Offensive diarrhoea, easily passed; sensitive to any changes of temperature with very offensive odours; not chilly. Consider Hepar Sulph for dental abscesses.

Also consider . . .

Calcarea Carbonica; Hepar Sulphurius Calcarea; Mercurius Solubilis; Pulsatilla; and other remedies according to notable symptoms.

Staphysagria (Staphisagria)

Usual abbreviation: **Staph**

 Better for breakfast

 Worse for repressed emotions

 Very sensitive to touch

 Worse if sleeps in afternoon

Remedy made from seeds of the Delphinium plant (licebane).

Key words

Lice. Anaemia. Indignation, wrongful accusation, insult, disappointment, humiliation. Rage. Trembling. Cystitis after coitus. Sweats. Easily offended. Pain-sensitive. Frontal headache affects eyeballs.

Possible precipitating situations

Lice. Disappointed in love. Victim of bullying, robbery or assault. Helpless indignation and rage without an outlet. Trauma from tissues being cut, swollen or stretched apart; stab wounds; surgical interventions; caesarian section. Excessive sexual intercourse. Childbirth, pregnancy.

Main signs and symptoms

General/physical

> Toothache.
> Headache (frontal) or stomach pain, after perceived or actual violation.
> Testes swollen from mumps.
> Anaemia.
> Pain follows use of sharp instruments; catheterization; laparoscopy.
> Diarrhoea, colic or travel sickness; after perceived violation.
> Trembling and shaking.
> Painful cystitis symptoms when not urinating. Prostatitis.
> Urinary stress incontinence, frequency, pressure and burning sensation.
> Post-operative pain and infections of pelvic, urinary and sexual systems.
> Lice of the head or pubic area (treat with tincture overnight).
> ■ Styes; sunken, dry eyes.

Mental/emotional

> ■ Hypersensitive to pain, and to criticism or imagined slights.
> Unexpressed feelings of humiliation; anger; indignation. Sense of injustice.
> Craves sweets, alcohol, meat. Dislike for dairy foods.
> Reactive insomnia.

Modalities

Worse: for negative emotional outbursts; for cold or cold drinks; for touch or pressure on site of pain; for tobacco; for missing a meal; after afternoon nap.

Better: for warmth and relaxation; for breakfast; if learns to resist when asked favours would rather refuse, rather than build resentments.

Look for different remedy if . . .

Able to express anger openly; screaming with the pain; sighing, yawning and suppressing grief which is worse for sympathy. Capricious mental states. Hormonal imbalances and uncharacteristic indifference to needs of others.

Also consider . . .

Chamomilla; Ignatia Amara; Sepia; and other remedies according to notable symptoms.

Sulphur (Sulphur)

Usual abbreviation: Sul

 Better for warm/dry weather

 Better for fresh air

Craves spicy, sweet foods

Hot feet, especially at night

Remedy made from Brimstone, the mineral Flowers of Sulphur.

Key words

Unkempt appearance. Burning; itching. Offensive odours. Head feels constricted. Congestion. Slouches when erect, slumps when sitting. Catarrh. Red face, red lips. thirsts for water. Worse for bathing; better for fresh air. Top of head hot. Often wears sandals.

Possible precipitating situations

Overeating or overexertion. Bathing. Becoming too hot or too cold. Menopausal hot flushes. Change of weather from cool to hot. *NB: To treat eczema symptoms consult a professional homeopath. All chronic condition symptoms can be seriously aggravated by amateur prescribing.*

Main signs and symptoms

General/physical

Burning and itching anywhere.

Redness, sometimes in spots; red face, and red lips; dry and cracked.

Offensive odours from breath, any and all excretions. Bad taste in mouth.

■ Sweats copiously. Dislikes washing.

Dry and scaly skin.

■ Scruffy appearance of which they are unaware and uncaring.

Cannot bear airless room.

Headaches as if wearing too tight a hat.

■ Eyes sticky in the morning but cannot bear to wash them.

Eyes sore, gritty, burning, red.

Swollen glands.

Tongue furred white with red tip and edges.

Great thirst for water.

Hunger mid-morning.

Urgent diarrhoea in early morning. Swollen abdomen. Constipation.

■ Hair loss when pregnant.

Hot feet, especially at night; may wear sandals in all weathers.

Mental/emotional

A conceptualizer, but not a realizer, of numerous schemes. Vivid imagination.

Fascinated with religious, theological and philosophical questions.

■ Impatient, irritable, lazy, quarrelsome, self-centred.

Ever-questioning child who becomes an impractically imaginative adult.

- Desires sweets and highly seasoned, fatty foods. Mid-morning hunger.
- Dislikes eggs, meat and strong cheeses.

Modalities

Worse: for warmth which increases itching; for bathing; in the early morning and at night; for stuffy rooms; for standing.
Better: for fresh air; movement; dry, warm weather; for short naps.

Look for different remedy if . . .

Swellings during the initial stage of illness; very chilly; of tidy appearance; unimaginative; pale faced; no offensive odours; treating chronic conditions. NB: most remedies have sulphur-like symptoms so check carefully for supporting proof before selecting. Often prescribed to follow acute treatment.

Also consider . . .

Aconite; Nux Vomica; and other remedies according to notable symptoms.

Every care has been taken in the preparation of this Materia Medica and Repertory. Nonetheless if errors or omissions have occurred, I apologize and will correct them for future reprints if brought to my attention.

APPENDIX 1
A CASE STUDY:
JANE DOE

A tearful Jane Doe went to see her homeopath complaining of feeling utterly exhausted and depressed. Invited to take a seat, Jane slumped into a chair, coughing loudly. The homeopath asked how she could help, noting as she did so the general appearance of this patient; a somewhat overweight young woman with coarse hair, a sallow complexion and a posture which suggested exhaustion. There was also a hint of stale sweat about her.

Jane explained her problem. 'I am so tired, I do not know how to get through the day sometimes, and the evenings are even worse. I just seem to have no energy or interest in anything these days. The least little thing reduces me to tears sometimes, but I couldn't tell you why. My husband keeps telling me to see a doctor, but I don't want to be put on antidepressants. It is as if I have no strength left in my body; what is wrong with me?

The homeopath asked Jane a few questions and discovered that Jane was also experiencing sick headaches, and felt faint quite often. Her feet felt cold most of the time and her skin had become itchy, often with a visible rash. In addition she had sometimes experienced the sensation of pins and needles prickling her skin. Asked about her menstrual cycle, Jane confided that it had become erratic and troublesome for the first time in her life. At the start of menstruation she was experiencing painful cramps and low back pain with a heavy dragging sensation which added to her general feeling of misery and exhaustion. Quite often she found it impossible to work on such days and she was becoming worried that she might lose her job if her sickness record did not improve. Asked if she had noticed that anything made her feel better, Jane replied, 'Funnily enough, if I simply have to do physical work, or chase about after my children, even when I don't feel like it, I do feel better. I even joined an exercise class for a while, and that did help, but then the class closed and I couldn't be bothered to find another one. Oh yes, one more thing; I always feel better when I have eaten. If I get too hungry or cold I feel miserable. I hate the winter, but what can you do?'

The homeopath noted all the symptoms and added a note of her own observations. Based on many years of experience, she suspected the tell-tale signs of a sepia type, but as a professional, she first checked the symptom picture with the repertory and the homeopathic materia medica before confirming this diagnosis. She then determined and administered the appropriate potency of the remedy sepia. She explained to Jane the principles of homeopathy, how to keep and handle the remedy and which foods and other substances to avoid when taking it, especially immediately before and after doing so. She also reminded Jane that she must stop taking the remedy as soon as the symptom picture abated or changed. Finally she made an appointment to follow up the results of the treatment.

APPENDIX 2
GLOSSARY

aggravation A temporary intensification of symptoms, a sign that the remedy is well selected to trigger a cure. Aggravation is more noticeable in the treatment of chronic conditions rather than acute ones, when it may occur for days or weeks before being replaced by a sense of greater well being. There may be progressive stages of aggravation in chronic cases, as layers of suppression are released. See Hering's Laws of Cure.

allopathy Samuel Hahnemann created the term to described conventional medicine and distinguish it from homeopathy (From the Greek words *allo* – other than or different from and *pathos* – suffering). Sometimes referred to as *contraria contraris*, the treatment of opposites with opposites.

antidote Any agent or experience which interferes with the effectiveness of a homeopathic remedy. It may also interfere with an unwanted condition.

case, taking the The meticulous gathering of information relative to the specific person who is experiencing dis-ease, regarded as essential by the homeopath for determining the treatment required. A lengthy interview employing special techniques for this purpose.

centesimal Division by hundreds.

chronic A recurrent condition, usually accompanied with a gradual deterioration in general health, which will not abate without intervention.

constitution The individual picture of a person's health shaped by the influence of lifestyle and environment, past illnesses and treatments, inherited predispositions, present situation and diet.

constitutional treatment A remedy dictated by the individual constitution intended to boost the natural, innate tendency towards health and entirely remove the affliction rather than to diminish specific symptoms of dis-ease. The encouragement of natural powers of regeneration.

decimal   Division by tenths.

dis-ease, (disease)   An interruption of the natural state of harmonious balance of an individual. This may affect physical, mental or emotional well-being, singly, together or all three at once.

drug picture   Synopsis of all the bodily changes – physical, mental and emotional – a substance is capable of inducing in a healthy individual. The substance can cure the same symptoms as it produces.

dynamization   *see* potentization/succussion.

essential nature   Essence, defining core of being.

Hahnemann, Samuel (13 April 1755–2 July 1843)   Founder of modern homeopathy.

health   A sense of well-being, equilibrium and vitality secondary to a balanced vital force which allows normal functioning.

Hering's Laws of Cure   The principles of the curative process, first described by Constantine Hering (1800–1880). (1) Healing proceeds from inner to outer, from most vital to less vital organs, using the shortest available route. (2) Healing occurs in a reverse of the order that dis-ease symptoms occurred: the last to appear will be the first to go. (3) Healing proceeds from above to below; from head to foot. The reverse of these principles would lead to death.

homeopathy   Medical treatment of like with like in order to stimulate a reflexive cure.

homeoprophylaxis   Homeopathic treatment based on constitional type, intended to boost the vital force while well rather than address a present health imbalance.

infinitesimal dose   (*see* **minimum dose**).

Laws of Cure   The laws of cure are the normal stages of the healing process.

materia medica   An alphabetical list of remedy descriptions, their origins and properties sometimes with instructions on dosage and use. May be for allopathic or homeopathic prescribing, though the basic philosophy underpinning each differs considerably.

miasm   A barrier to health which may be hereditary or acquired as a result of past dis-ease. Creates an obstacle to the healing process.

minimum dose (*also* **infinitesimal dose**)   The smallest application of a potentized remedy to trigger the healing process. In homeopathy there are actually no doses, as each application of a remedy is entire and not a fraction of the whole, though potencies vary.

modalities   That which affects symptoms to become better or worse, such as heat, fresh air, sitting. Often noted symbolically by: > (is better for) < (is worse for).

mother tincture   Designated by the symbol ø. Substance in an alcohol or double distilled water solution, the starting material for producing homeopathically prepared remedies.

Organon, The   Samuel Hahnemann's published description of his pioneering work and the philosophy of homeopathy, *The Organon of the Healing Arts*. Organon = the means.

polycrest   A remedy which is effective for many different conditions having been found to produce a wide range of symptoms in provings.

potency   The strength a remedy has, dependent on how many times it has been diluted and succussed.

potentization   The energizing preparation of a homeopathic remedy. Potentization describes how the mother tincture is rendered more homeopathically effective by the process of succussion; repeated dilution and succussion (vibration). Potency is the strength of the resulting remedy.

provers   Courageous and dedicated human volunteers who systematically test substances to discover their homeopathic values.

proving   Discovering the symptom picture of a substance by systematically testing on healthy human volunteers. The symptoms a substance induces in a healthy person can effect a cure in a sick person. Provings are not carried out on animals because communication of the experience is an essential element.

remedy   The name given to a homeopathically prepared medicine.

remedy picture   The list of the symptoms of all kinds known to be produced by a substance when given to a healthy human.

repertory   An index of symptoms noted in the homeopathic materia medica, listed alphabetically together with the likely remedies associated with them.

repertory grid   A graph used to simplify the selection of the correct remedy from the symptoms gathered when taking the case.

repertory list   A list prepared from the case notes for ease of analysis.

Similia similibus curentur: *Let Like Be Treated With Like*   The law of similars.

Similimum   The remedy which most closely matches the symptoms an individual exhibits (and not similar causes of disease, as is the case with allopathy).

succussion   When potentizing a homeopathic remedy the solution is shaken or banged vigorously at each successive dilution. This is usually performed by machines today, as hand diluting and succussing a single remedy to the required potency may take weeks.

symptom   A change or perceived change to the normal physical, emotional or mental state which indicates the body is reacting to stress or injury.

symptom picture   An overview of all a patient's symptoms noted when case taking. The symptom picture is compared with a list of remedy pictures to find the nearest overall match.

tincture   *see* **mother tincture**

trituration   Insoluble substances which cannot be diluted in alcohol or distilled water are made soluble by grinding with a mortar and pestle, a process called trituration.

vital force   The life principle, energy or motivating force, the organizing principle within all living beings which can be stimulated to effect a cure.

> Better for; symbol used to denote a modality which affects symptoms.

< Worse for; symbol used to denote a modality which affects symptoms.

APPENDIX 3
SAMPLE CASE NOTES

(The following is not an actual symptom picture, but is used to illustrate the sorts of points to consider. A real case may or may not include all these particular variables.)

Make a note of the date and time of the consultation. (Do not rely on memory to record details later.) Name and date of birth of the patient. The current age of the patient. The reason given for seeking help, for example, severe cold, measles, insomnia, minor injury and so on. Make preliminary observations on first meeting. Question the patient concerning changes to physical, mental, emotional, general, environmental and family conditions. The following list is a reminder of the points which will help to identify the case and the sort of questions you may ask.

How would you describe the problem?

What symptoms have you noticed?

Where is the problem located? Is it always in the same place?

Has this happened before? How did you recover before?

Is it a recurring problem? Have you taken medical advice?

■ Are your moods affected?

Is it made better or worse by anything that you have noticed?

Describe the type of pain.

How does it affect your emotional or mental well being?

Your initial observations

For example, scruffy appearance to hair and clothes, smells of stale sweat, agitated. Note the overall sense of well being, the severity and location of each symptom, and how the person describes it themselves.

Overall

Emotions: tearful, manic, depressed, happy, sad, angry, afraid, and so on. Mental symptoms: forgetful, unfocused, confused, alert, over stimulated. General symptoms: feels exhausted.

Symptoms

- Head: feels larger than normal, throbs with movement.
- Hair: dry, splitting at the ends, patchy loss.
- Face: sore lips, flushed cheeks, patches of dry skin.
- Nose: occasional dripping, persistent tickle. Red around nostrils.
- Mouth: gum ulcers very painful. Furred tongue. Metallic taste.
- Ears: left ear has hearing loss. Sudden onset. Both ears itching, burning.
- Eyes: whites tinged yellow, puffy eyelids. Sight blurred, worse in sunlight.
- Throat: intensely sore. Inflamed tonsils. Dry, difficulty swallowing.
- Neck: stiffness on turning, painful swollen glands.
- Chest: pains radiating to the back, shortness of breath, gradual onset.
- Back: low back pain, sharp pain between shoulders.
- Arms/legs: heaviness, dull ache, localized numbness.
- Skin: dry, scaly.
- Bowels: recent constipation, now diarrhoea, green smelly.
- Urination: frequent, with a burning sensation.
- Abdomen: excessive gas, flatulence. Relieves temporarily.

■ Stomach: loss of appetite, vomits after food.
■ Sleep: frequent waking. Unable to return to sleep.
■ Dreams: nightmares.
■ Made better by or worse by which modalities?

worse for (<)	*better for* (>)
<fresh air	>touch
<sitting/standing/lying/movement	>applied heat/cold
<weather conditions	
<time of day	
<eating/drinking	
<being covered/uncovered	

■ Environmental influences: have there been changes to your personal, family, home or working life recently? (Enquire whether any recent emotional stress factors: bereavement, divorce, stress, anger, house move, redundancy, more responsibilities, becoming a parent, weather conditions difficult, robbery or attack, benefited from an inheritance, promoted, learned a relative is ill, exposure to chemical hazards, started or stopped smoking or drinking alcohol, used illicit drugs.) Have you recently started, stopped or changed a prescribed medicine? Can you think of any changes affecting your life at the moment?

APPENDIX 4
ACTION CHECKLIST

1 Assess the severity of the complaint and your suitability to treat the patient. Call emergency help if indicated.
2 Refer the patient to a professional homeopath or conventional practitioner if treatment is beyond the scope of this book or your abilities.
3 Interview and take the case history if you are to proceed with treatment.
4 Decide on the key symptoms and enter them on a separate list or grid. Look up the remedies associated with these symptoms in the repertory. Add them to your list/grid. Analyse and score the results to refine the selection of the remedy.
5 If several remedies seem indicated, read the remedy picture for each one in the homeopathic materia medica to eliminate those less well matched to the whole symptom picture and find the best possible match.
6 Decide the correct potency, frequency and dosage of the remedy and prescribe.
7 Give advice concerning the risk of contamination causing antidoting, and general lifestyle changes which might be an aid to health.
8 Keep a dated record of the questionnaire, your analysis and the recommended remedy, and prescription details with your suggestions for lifestyle changes, if any.
9 Allow time for the remedy to have an effect and arrange a time to assess results. If an acute situation, assess and re-administer as necessary.

10 Record the results, including changed symptoms which alter the overall picture and may require different prescribing. Note aggravation as well as increased well being. Note if the decision not to act improves symptoms as well as when intervention does.

APPENDIX 5
COMPLEMENTARY
THERAPIES

Therapies such as acupuncture and aromatherapy are excluded from this list because, though excellent, they also work on the body's energy patterns and could obscure the symptom picture needed for homeopathy.

Counselling
Cranial osteopathy
Dietitian
Massage

Osteopathy
Physiotherapy
Psychotherapy
Reflexology

Counselling

May be found helpful where current, or deep-seated problems are affecting emotional, social or psychological well being. Specialist counsellors are available to help with many specific issues, such as bereavement counselling; family dynamics; financial matters; marital guidance; religious beliefs; sexual health and victim support. Consult a trained counsellor who receives continued support through membership of a professional body. A professional homeopath can also treat issues involving the mind and emotions, which are believed to have deep-seated organic origins.

Cranial osteopathy

This remarkable therapy can help relieve pain associated with skeletal misalignment or injury when other therapies are ill advised. By manipulation of particular areas of the head, relief may be brought to distant areas of the body which are too painful to be touched or manipulated directly.

Dietitian

Diet plays a vital role in the maintenance of health. A professional dietitian will advise how to attain a healthy body weight; will assess deficiencies in your diet, and advise how to correct them; suggest alternatives to poorly tolerated foods and give advice on the foods to avoid in the case of a specific sensitivity; and may advise which foods antidote homeopathic remedies. Advice on eating disorders is available from specialists.

Massage

Massage is well known as a wonderful way to release stress, but in the hands of a professional may also be the means of stimulating sluggish body systems. Working on the soft tissues, muscles and skin, massage may gently restore or improve function to injured or incapacitated areas of the body. There are many variants of massage technique available.

Osteopathy

Osteopathy aims to achieve the correct alignment of bones, muscles, ligaments and nerves by manipulation of the spine and individual joints using the principles of medicine and engineering. Check the register of qualified osteopaths for a qualified practitioner.

Physiotherapy

Physiotherapy is widely accepted and available as an adjunct to orthodox medicine. It involves the manipulation of body parts to restore or improve functioning, mobility and the feeling of well being.

Psychotherapy

Psychotherapy addresses emotional and psychological issues where mental dis-equilibrium affects the whole person. Imbalance often involves a sense of identity, such as an eating disorder; a personality disorder; present or past traumas. There are very many theoretical beliefs and methodologies, but most take the approach that we have an unconscious, with or without a spiritual dimension, and interaction with it can lead to the restoration of healthy equilibrium. A professional homeopath can also treat issues involving the mind and emotions, which are believed to have deep seated organic origins.

Reflexology

Areas of the feet, particularly the soles and sides, are believed to correspond to the organs of the body. Reflexology involves the massage of specific points to diagnose areas of dis-ease, and promote healthy functioning. The massage of the affected area of the foot continues until pain or sensitivity subsides.

APPENDIX 6
USEFUL ADDRESSES

While every attempt has been made to verify these addresses at the time of publication, their continued accuracy cannot be guaranteed.

Australia

Australian Association of Professional Homeopaths, 80 Essendon Road, Anstead, Brisbane. Tel: 3202 6517

Australian Homeopathic Association, PO Box 82, Gladesville 2111, 243 Victoria Road, Gladesville, Sydney. Tel: 9879 0049

The Australian Federation of Homeopaths, Suite 14, London Court, Perth. Tel: 9325 2579

Brauer Biotherapies (Pharmacy), 1 Para Road, Gin Forest, Tanunda, South Australia 5352. Tel: 9298 9071

Homeopathic Pharmacy, 387 Payneham Road, Marden, Adelaide. Tel: 8362 2729

New Zealand

The Auckland College of Classical Homeopathy, PO Box 19502, Auckland 7. Tel: 0-9-828 9200

The NZ Hahnemann College of Homeopathy, 6 Poronui Street, Mount Eden, Auckland. Tel: AK 638 8853

The NZ Institute of Classical Homeopathy, PO Box 7232, Wellesley Street, Auckland. Tel: 424 5844

The Wellington College of Homeopathy Clinic, 99 Main Road, Tawa, Wellington. Tel: WN-232 7942

South Africa

Health and Homeopathic Products, 4 Heathway Shopping Centre, DF Malan Drive, Blackheath, PO Box 35758, Northcliffe, Johannesburg. Tel: 678 5811

Homeopathic and Health Centre, 53 Anthony Street, 13 Canford Park, Umgeni Park, Durban. Tel: 84 9177

Homeopathic Laboratories, Clothing Centre, 69 Sivewright Avenue, Doornfontein, Box 6071, Johannesburg. Tel: 402 3409

Natura Homeopathic Laboratory, 18e Street, 7 Hazelwood, Pretoria, SA. Tel: 346 1230

The Peace + Love Foundation, 152 Blackburn Road, Red Hill, Durban. Tel: 84 5713

United Kingdom

Homeopathic training for the Medically Qualified

The British Homoeopathic Association, 27a Devonshire Street, London W1N 1RJ. Tel: 0171 935 2163 (founded 1902) Registered as a charity. Members entitled to use MFHOM as accreditation. Can supply information on postgraduate training, lists of doctors who practise homeopathy, National Health Service hospitals and outreach clinics. Well stocked library available to members.

The Faculty of Homoeopathy, The Royal London Homoeopathic Hospital, London WC1N 3HR. Tel: 0171 837 9469/3091 ext 7285. Professional organization for medical homeopathy. Trains doctors, veterinarians, dental surgeons and pharmacists, so long as they have qualifications which can be registered with General Medical Council, Royal College of Veterinary Surgeons, General Dental Council or Royal Pharmaceutical Society.

The Homoeopathic Society, Hahnemann House, 2 Powis Place, Great Ormond Street, London WC1N 3HT. Tel: 0171 837 3297. Produces a magazine, *Health & Homeopathy*, by subscription.

Homeopathic Physicians Teaching Group, 28 Beaumont Street, Oxford OX1 2NP. Tel: 01865 552706

The United Kingdom Homeopathic Medical Association,
6 Livingstone Road, Gravesend, Kent. DA12 5DZ.
Tel: 01474 560336

Homeopathic training without prior medical qualifications

England

College of Homoeopathy, Regent's College, Inner Circle, Regent's Park, London NW1 4NS. Tel: 0171 487 7416

College of Homoeopathy Teaching Clinic, 26 Clarendon Rise, London, SE13 5EY. Tel: 0181 852 6573

College of Practical Homoeopathy (London), Oakwood House, 422 Hackney Road, London, E2 7SY. Tel: 0171 613 5468

College of Practical Homoeopathy (Midlands),
186 Wolverhampton Street, Dudley, West Midlands DY1 3AD.
Tel: 01384 233664

Hahnemann College of Homeopathy, 342 Barking Road, Plaistow, London, E13 8HI. Tel: 0171 476 7263. Treatment available by students of the college.

Hahnemann College of Homeopathy, 243 The Broadway, Southall, Middlesex UB1 1NF. Tel: 0181 574 4281

London College of Classical Homoeopathy, Morley College, 61 Westminster Bridge Road, London SE1 7HT. Tel: 0171 928 6199

London College of Classical Homoeopathy, 32 Welbeck Street, London W1M. Tel: 0171 487 4322 or 4320

North West College of Homoeopathy, 23 Wilbraham Road, Fallowfield, Manchester M14 6FB. Tel: 0161 257 2445

Northern College of Homoeopathic Medicine, First Floor, Swinburne House, Swinburne Street, Gateshead, Tyne and Wear NE8 1AX. Tel: 0191 490 0276

School of Homoeopathy, Yondercott House, Uffculme, Devon EX15 3DR. Tel: 01873 856872

The Society of Homoeopaths, 2 Artizan Road, Northampton NN1 4HU. Tel: 01604 621400. The main professional organization for non-medical homoeopathy in the UK. Members entitled to use RSHOM as accreditation.

Ireland

The Irish Society of Homeopaths, 35–37 Dominick Street, Galway. Tel: 091 565040, The equivalent professional body to the Society of Homeopaths in England.

Herbal Homoeopathic Clinic, Natural Remedies, Eagle House, Sidmonton Avenue, Bray, Co Wicklow. Tel: 01 286 6280

The Irish Medical Homeopathic Association, 115 Morehampton Road, Donnybrook 4. Tel: Donnybrook 2697768

Morehampton Pharmacy, 79 Morehampton Road, Dublin 4. Tel: 01 668 7103

Nelson's Homeopathic Pharmacy, 15 Duke Street, Dublin 2. Tel: 01 679 0451

Scotland

The Scottish College of Homeopathy, 11 Lynedoch Place, Glasgow GA3 3AB. Tel: 0141 332 3917

The Faculty of Homeopathy, The Claremont Homeopathic Clinic, 11b North Claremont Street, Glasgow G3 7NR. Tel: 0141 331 0393

Wales

School of Homoeopathy, 8 Kiln Road, Llanfoist, Abgergavenny, Gwent NP7 9NS. Tel: 01873 856872

Homeopathic hospitals

British Homoeopathic Hospital, Cotham Hill, Cotham, Bristol BS6 6JU. Tel: 0117 973 1231

Glasgow Homoeopathic Hospital, 1000 Great Western Road, Glasgow G12 0NR. Tel: 0141 211 1600

The Royal London Homoeopathic Hospital, Great Ormond Street, London WC1N 3HR. Tel: 0171 837 8833

Tunbridge Wells Homoeopathic Hospital, Church Road, Tunbridge Wells, Kent TN1 1JV. Tel: 01892 542977

Correspondence Training Courses

The School of Homoeopathy, Yondercott House, Uffculme, Devon EX15 3DR. Tel: 01873 856872

Suppliers of homeopathic books

Ainsworths Homeopathic Pharmacy, 36 New Cavendish Street, London W1M 7LH. Lists available. Order by phone or in person. Tel: 018833 40332.

The British Homoeopathic Association, 27a Devonshire Street, London W1N 1RJ. Tel: 0171 935 2163. Also has a mail order service with lists available.

East Asia Company, 101-103 Camden High Street, London NW1. Tel: 0171 388 5783/6704

Minerva Homeopathic Books, 173 Fulham Palace Road, London W6. Tel: 0171 385 1361

Homeopathic research

The Homeopathic Trust for Research and Education, 2 Powis Place, London WC1N 3HT. Tel: 0171 837 9469. Fax: 0171 278 7900

Suppliers of Homeopathic Remedies

Ainsworth Homeopathic Pharmacy, 36 New Cavendish Street, London W1M 7LH. Tel: 0171 935 5330

Bumblebees Natural Remedies, 35 Brecknock Road, London N7 6AD. Tel: 0171 267 3884 or 0171 670 1936

Buxton and Grant, 176 Whiteladies Road, Bristol BS8 2XU. Tel: 0117 973 5025

Galen Homeopathic Pharmacy, Lewel Mill, West Stafford, Dorchester, Dorset DT2 8AN. Tel: 01305 263996

Goulds, 14 Crowndale Road, London NW1 1TT. Tel: 0171 388 4752

Helios Homeopathic Pharmacy, 97 Camden Road, Tunbridge Wells, Kent TN1 2QR. Tel: 01892 537254 and 536393. Fax: 01892 546850

National Homeopathic Service, 191a Kentish Town Road, London NW5. Tel: 0171 482 0432

Nelson and Co Ltd, Customer Services, 5 Endeavour Way, London SW19 9UH. Tel: 0181 946 8527

Nelson's Homeopathy & Bach Remedies, 73 Duke Street, London W1M 6BY. Tel: 0171 629 3118 and 0171 495 2404

Noma (Complex Homeopathy) Ltd, Unit 3, 1–16 Holybrook Road, Upper Shierly, Southampton SO16 6RB. Tel: 01703 770513

United States of America

American Institute of Homeopathy, 925 East 17th Avenue, Denver, Colorado 80218–1407. Tel: (303) 321 4105

Homeopathic Educational Services, 2124b Kittredge Street, Berkeley, CA 94704. Tel: (510) 649-0294. Fax: (510) 649-1955

Homeopathy for Health, 422 n. Earl Road, Moses Lake, Wa. Toll free for US and Canadian customers 1-800-390-9970 (1-509-766-0182) 8am to 5pm Pacific Standard Time.

The National Centre for Homeopathy, 801 North Fairfax Street, Suite 306, Alexandria, Virginia 22314. Tel: 703 548 7790 for newsletter and educational programs concerning homeopathy. Can also advise of homeopaths, medical and professional, practising in your locality.

US remedy suppliers

Longevity Pure Medicines, a division of Lacausa inc. 9595 Wilshire Blvd, Suite 502 Beverly Hills, CA 90212. Tel: (310) 273 7423

For remedy manufacturers in US contact:

The Homeopathic Pharmacopoeia of the United States, PO Box 80185, Valley Forge, PA 19484. Tel: (610) 783 5124/0987

International Foundation for Homeopathy (IFH), PO Box 7, Edmonds, WA 98020. Tel: (206) 776 4147

BIBLIOGRAPHY

Blackie, Margery. *The Challenge of Homoeopathy*, Unwin Hyman, 1981

Boericke, William, MD. *Materia Medica with Repertory*, Indian edition, Homeopathic Publications, New Delhi, 1927

Castro, Miranda. *The Complete Homeopathy Handbook – A guide to everyday health care*, Macmillan, London, 1990

Coulter, Harris L. *Homoeopathic science and modern medicine: the physics of healing with microdoses*, North Atlantic Books, 1987

Dannheisser, Ilana and Edwards, Penny. *Homeopathy. An illustrated guide*, Element Books Ltd, Dorset, 1998

Garion-Hutchings, Nigel and Susan. *The Concise Guide to Homoeopathy*, Element Books Ltd, Dorset, 1993

Hahnemann, Samuel (trans. William Boericke, MD). *Organon of Medicine*, 6th edition, *Homoeopathic Publications*, New Delhi, 1921

Kent, James Tyler, AM, MD. *Lectures on Homoeopathic Materia Medica*, Indian edition, Homeopathic Publications, New Delhi, 1911

Kent, James Tyler, AM, MD, *Lectures on homoeopathic philosophy*, B Jain Publishers PVT. Ltd, New Delhi, reprint edition 1990

Kent, James Tyler, AM, MD, *Repertory of the homoeopathic materia medica*, Indian edition, reprinted from 6th American edition, Homeopathic Publications, New Delhi, 1945

Maceoin, Beth. *Homoeopathy and the menopause*, Thorsons/ Harper Collins, 1995

Nash, EB, MD. *Leaders in homoeopathic therapeutics*, 6th edition, National Homoeopathic Pharmacy, New Delhi, c. 1915

Roberts, Herbert A, MD. *The principles and art of cure by homoeopathy*, Indian books and Periodicals Syndicate, New Delhi, 1936

Smith, Dr Trevor, MA, MB, BCHIR, DPM, MFHOM. *Homeopathy for pregnancy and nursing mothers*, Insight editions, Worthing, Sussex, 1993

Tyler, Dr ML, MD, LRCP, LRCS, LRFPS. *Homoeopathic Drug Pictures*, B Jain Publishers PVT. Ltd, New Delhi, 1980

Vithoulkas, George. *Homoeopathy, Medicine of the New Man*, Thorsons Publishing Group, 1979

HOMEOPATHY AND THE WORLD WIDE WEB

Colorado Institute For Classical Homeopathy – a training program in homeopathic medicine.
http://www.coloradohomeopathy.org

For conventional and alternative advice at all levels:
http://www.healthy.net

For first aid advice:
http://www.prairienet.org/~atumn/firsaid/

Healthworld online – healthworld is a large site providing access to a broad range of alternative medicine information, organizations, services, and products.
http://www.healthy.com

Homeopathic Association of Naturopathic Physicians (HANP)
http://www.healthy.net/hanp

The Homeopathy Home Page – this website provides a listing of various homeopathic resources and websites throughout the world. You can also subscribe, without cost, to a homeopathic discussion group, or you can access various past discussion topics by searching their table of contents.
http://www.homeopathyhome.com

Homeopathic Links (A Homeopathic Journal) – an excellent homeopathic journal for serious students or practitioners of homeopathy
http://www.antenna.nl/homeolinks

The National Center for Homeopathy/NCH – the NCH is the leading homeopathic organization in the United States. This site includes articles plus a searchable directory for homeopaths in US.
http://www.homeopathic.org

New England Journal of Homeopathy – an excellent journal for serious students and practitioners of homeopathy.
http://www.nesh.com/main/nejh.html

Online Training in Hahnemannian Homeopathy – this is a site for serious students of classical homeopathy. Developed by a master homeopath, David Little, this site provides detailed instruction in Hahnemann's homeopathy.
http://www.ioa.com/home/davehart/little.html

Will Taylor, MD/Homeopath and educator – a lot of good information for serious students and practitioners of homeopathy, with a primary focus of classical homeopathy.
http://www.simillibus.com/remedyoftheweek.html

INDEX